Dynamic Patterns of Brain Cell Assemblies

A report

based on an NRP Work Session
held May 14-16, 1972

and updated by participants

Aharon Katzir Katchalsky and Vernon Rowland (Co-Chairmen)

Report by

Vernon Rowland
Case Western Reserve University
School of Medicine
Cleveland, Ohio

and

Robert Blumenthal
National Cancer Institute
National Institutes of Health
Bethesda, Maryland

Yvonne M. Homsy
Writer-Editor

This book was first published as Volume 12, No. 1, March 1974, of the *Neurosciences Research Program Bulletin.*

This book was printed and bound in the United States of America

ISBN 0 262 11056 3
Library of Congress catalog card number: 74–6982

CONTENTS

4

PARTICIPANTS

Dr. W. Ross Adey
Department of Anatomy
University of California
   School of Medicine
The Center for the Health Sciences
Los Angeles, California 90024

Dr. Michael V.L. Bennett
Department of Anatomy
920 Kennedy Center
Albert Einstein College of Medicine
Bronx, New York 10461

Dr. Floyd E. Bloom
Laboratory of Neuropharmacology
National Institute of Mental Health
Saint Elizabeth's Hospital
Washington, D.C. 20032

Dr. Robert Blumenthal
Laboratory of Theoretical Biology
National Cancer Institute
Building 10-4B50
Bethesda, Maryland 20014

Dr. Theodore H. Bullock
Department of Neurosciences
University of California, San Diego
   School of Medicine
La Jolla, California 92037

Dr. Eduardo Eidelberg
Division of Neurobiology
Barrow Neurological Institute
350 West Thomas Road
Phoenix, Arizona 85013

Dr. Rafael Elul
Department of Anatomy
University of California
   School of Medicine
The Center for the Health Sciences
Los Angeles, California 90024

Dr. John H. Ferguson
Division of Neurology
Case Western Reserve University
   School of Medicine
2065 Adelbert Road
Cleveland, Ohio 44106

Dr. Walter J. Freeman
Department of Physiology-Anatomy
University of California
2549 Life Science Building
Berkeley, California 94720

Dr. Robert Galambos
Department of Neurosciences
University of California, San Diego
   School of Medicine
La Jolla, California 92037

Dr. Robert G. Grossman
Department of Neurological Surgery
Albert Einstein College of Medicine
1300 Morris Park Avenue
Bronx, New York 10461

Dr. Aharon Katzir Katchalsky
Polymer Department
Weizmann Institute of Science
Rehovot, Israel

Dr. Frank Morrell
Department of Neurology
Rush Medical College
Rush-Presbyterian-St. Luke's
   Medical Center
Chicago, Illinois 60612

Dr. Daniel Pollen
Neurosurgical Service
Massachusetts General Hospital
12 Fruit Street
Boston, Massachusetts 02114

Dr. Dominick P. Purpura
Department of Anatomy
903 Kennedy Center
Albert Einstein College of Medicine
Bronx, New York 10461

Dr. Wilfrid Rall
Mathematical Research Branch
National Institute of Arthritis
    and Metabolic Diseases
Building 31, Room 9A17
Bethesda, Maryland 20014

Dr. Vernon Rowland
Department of Psychiatry
Case Western Reserve University
    School of Medicine
2040 Abington Road
Cleveland, Ohio 44106

Dr. Francis O. Schmitt
Neurosciences Research Program
165 Allandale Street
Jamaica Plain Station
Boston, Massachusetts 02130

Dr. Otto H. Schmitt
Department of Electrical Engineering
University of Minnesota
Minneapolis, Minnesota 55455

Dr. L. E. Scriven
Department of Chemical Engineering
    and Materials Science
University of Minnesota
151 Chemical Engineering Building
Minneapolis, Minnesota 55455

George G. Somjen
Department of Physiology
    and Pharmacology
Duke University
Durham, North Carolina 27710

Dr. W. Alden Spencer
Department of Neurobiology
    and Behavior
Public Health Research Institute
    of City of New York
New York, New York 10016

Dr. William H. Sweet
Neurological Service
Massachusetts General Hospital
12 Fruit Street
Boston, Massachusetts 02114

Dr. Hendrik Van der Loos
Institut d'Anatomie Normale
Université de Lausanne
    Ecole de Médecine
9 Rue du Bugnon
Ch 1011 Lausanne, Switzerland

Dr. Anthonie Van Harreveld
Division of Biology
California Institute of Technology
1201 E. California Boulevard
Pasadena, California 91109

Dr. Paul A. Weiss
Professor Emeritus
The Rockefeller University
New York, New York 10021

Dr. Frederic G. Worden
Neurosciences Research Program
165 Allandale Street
Jamaica Plain Station
Boston, Massachusetts 02130

Dr. Yehoshua Zeevi
Department of Engineering
    and Applied Physics
Harvard University
Cambridge, Massachusetts 02138

Note: NRP Work Session summaries are reviewed and revised by participants prior to publication.

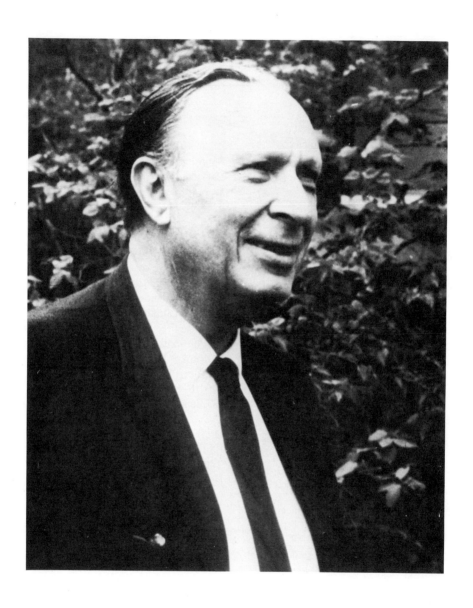

AHARON KATZIR KATCHALSKY

September 15, 1914 – May 30, 1972

NRP Associate 1962 – 1972

I. FOREWORD

In recent years Aharon Katchalsky became deeply interested in the theory of dynamic patterns, dissipative structures, and other nonequilibrium phenomena because of their significance for theoretical chemistry and for life science, particularly developmental biology and neurobiology. At successive meetings of Associates of the Neurosciences Research Program since 1962, he reported recent advances in the field and eloquently testified to his conviction that this area of biophysical chemistry may prove crucial for an understanding of molecular self-organization and development as well as brain function, which he conceived in a global, holistic frame of reference without primary consideration of brain architectonics and built-in neuronal circuitry mediating sensorimotor and other effects or processes.

The manifestations of brain function that lend themselves most obviously to analysis in terms of dynamic patterns are bioelectric phenomena, especially the direct current, steady potentials which have been demonstrated to show small but significant shifts as a function of neurophysiological and behavioral alterations. Discussions among NRP Associates, under the enthusiastic leadership of Aharon Katchalsky, led to the suggestion that a Work Session might be held along these lines. In due course, two planning sessions were held at which Drs. W.R. Adey, R. Blumenthal, T.H. Bullock, J. Ferguson, A. Katchalsky, V. Rowland, F.O. Schmitt, W.A. Spencer, and F.G. Worden were participants. It was recommended by them that, in addition to a discussion of the two major fields, i.e., physical chemistry of dynamic patterns and the neurophysiology of steady potential shifts as a function of neurophysiological and behavioral alterations (two poles at the ends of the conceptual spectrum), a variety of phenomena and theories, such as oscillatory fields, bioelectric pulse distribution, and pulse wave problems might also be included to help span the gap between the poles of chemical and neurobiological discussions. Despite the inhomogeneity and conceptual polarization between the thermodynamic and biophysical theory on the one hand and the phenomenology and basic neurophysiological theory of the functioning of the most complex mechanism known to man on the other hand, and the difficulties involved in bridging this gap, the consensus was that the Work Session should be undertaken, perhaps as the first of a possible series under the inspiring leadership of Aharon Katchalsky. Such theoretical and experimental advances, it was hoped, might fill in the gaps, produce closure, and establish a new hybrid between chemistry and neuroscience.

These expectant hopes were not to be realized, because only a few weeks after completion of this Work Session, Aharon Katchalsky's voice was stilled.* He would not articulate the proceedings of the Work Session in a synthesis uniquely his own, as he had planned. Nor would he carry forward in future Work Sessions the development of this promising aspect of neuroscience.

We are most grateful to Robert Blumenthal, a close colleague and student of Aharon Katchalsky and a member of the planning committee, for his willingness, as a labor of love, to write that portion of this report which would have been written by Aharon Katchalsky, in collaboration with the co-chairman of the Work Session, Vernon Rowland.

Thanks are also due to Manfred Eigen, Theodore H. Bullock, Jack Cowan, Stuart Kauffman, Richard Gordon, Tony Sastre, and L.E. Scriven for providing valuable material, discussion, and critical comments. John Ferguson provided the initial synopses of the contributions of the neurophysiologically oriented participants.

To the chief architect of this Work Session and the source of great inspiration to scientists interested in the vast spectrum from theoretical chemistry and biophysics to the functioning of the brain, our late colleague and friend, Aharon Katchalsky, this issue of the *NRP Bulletin* is affectionately dedicated.

Francis O. Schmitt
January, 1974

*Professor Katchalsky was slain by terrorists' bullets at Lod Airport, Tel Aviv, Israel, May 30, 1972.

II. CONCEPT OF DYNAMIC PATTERNS

Early History and Philosophy: A. Katchalsky

The concept of dynamic patterns embodies two basic features. First, systems are made up of a complex hierarchy of smaller and larger flow patterns in which "things" are self-maintaining features of the flows. This idea goes back to the Greek philosopher Heraclitus (540-480 B.C.; see Diels, 1909) whose conception was opposed by Democritus with his "reductionist" view, namely, that nature consists of "things" (atoms) in the void. Second, such flow patterns can undergo sudden transitions to new self-maintaining arrangements that will be relatively stable over time. The transformation of complex flow patterns into larger hierarchical patterns is saltatory, like the appearance of large crystals from small ones in a supersaturated solution.

The transitions are "symmetry breaking," a process which, according to the English philosopher Herbert Spencer (1880), is the first step in evolution. The concept of symmetry breaking is most adequately defined in Spencer's words: "Evolution is an integration of matter, and a concomitant dissipation of motion during which the matter passes from an indefinite incoherent homogeneity to a definite coherent heterogeneity, and during which the retained motion undergoes a parallel transformation." In other words, initially, energy, matter, and motion are symmetrically distributed among all the elements of a system permitting no organization or flows between groups of elements. The transition to a nonrandom distribution of energy, matter, and motion is "symmetry breaking" and has the characteristic generally understood by the terms pattern, form, or structure. An illustration of that idea was Spencer's observation that shellac varnish, made by dissolving shellac in light petroleum until it has the consistency of cream, will develop a honeycomb structure upon evaporation of the petroleum. The symmetry-breaking process is revealed by the formation of polygonal sections from the originally homogeneous film.

The concept of dynamic patterns and their hierarchical jumps is being applied in both the social and natural sciences. Platt (1970) extends the concept of sudden changes in organization to structures of personality, whole societies, and the field of ideas. He cites from *The Structure of Scientific Revolutions* (Kuhn, 1970) the jump transition in "weltanschauung" within a generation from the Ptolemaic to the Copernican system in astronomy, and the jump in the 1920's from classical to quantum mechanics in the field of physics. Multistable properties with jump transitions in perception have been approached by Attneave (1971), and Gestalt psychology has long emphasized this property. The restructuring of an individual personality may also take a sudden form as in the cases of flashes of understanding, learning a new skill, falling in love, or as in the conversion of St. Paul. In the area of whole societies, restructuring by sudden jump transitions becomes immediately obvious when one looks at the great social revolutions, and it may serve as the feature differentiating social revolution from evolution.

Examples of Dynamic Patterns in the Physical Sciences:
L. E. Scriven

A fundamental problem in the physical as well as the biological sciences is the origin of a dynamic pattern. In physical science it can be attacked at vulnerable points, i.e., systems that are simple enough to permit analysis both in physical and mathematical terms.

Dynamic patterns refer to those patterns that arise and are maintained by the dissipation or consumption of energy, such as traveling or standing waves generated in the air, on the surface of water, or in a vibrating violin string. They can be contrasted to static patterns, such as a stack of nesting chairs, a crystal, or a virus capsid.

The central question is: How does uniform matter, obeying physical principles, i.e., laws of conservation of momentum, matter, and energy, spontaneously develop regular patterns? In other words, how is it that a set of isotropic causes can give rise to anisotropic dynamic effects? This appears to be the root problem of morphogenesis; growing from it are the more widely encountered problems of how preexisting static structures influence dynamic patterns.

The first experiment that showed the appearance of structure through the dynamic interaction of flows was carried out by Bénard (1901) when he slowly heated the bottom of a petri dish containing spermaceti oil (see Figure 1, A and B). At a critical point, rings or cells of different refractive index appeared around the border of the liquid and then broke up into cylindrical structures that moved towards the center of the dish. Finally, the whole volume of liquid was filled with a honeycomb structure. A pure flow structure of this kind has no

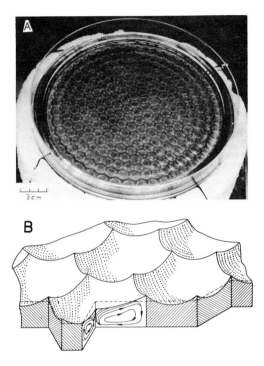

Figure 1. A. Development of Bénard cells in a dish of liquid heated uniformly from beneath. B. Schematic diagram of Bénard cells showing streamlines of flow within a single "honeycomb" cell. [Gmitro and Scriven, 1966]

covalent bonds to hold it together, nor is it a crystallization process; with insufficient or excessive heat flow, it disappears.

Lord Rayleigh (1916) interpreted the mechanism in the following way: heating a liquid from below gives rise to an unstable distribution of densities; this is compensated by a convectional flow that circulates between the hotter, buoyant fluid moving upwards and the colder, denser fluid moving downwards in columns. Bénard's cells were not caused by buoyancy mechanisms but by the surface tension variations along the free surface of the pool. Lord Rayleigh misinterpreted the physical phenomenon, but his theory was appropriate for those phenomena in which buoyancy is, indeed, the dominant process. This confusion illustrates an important property, namely, that two quite distinct mechanisms, one related to buoyancy and the other to surface tension, can give rise to the same dynamic pattern. A given pattern, therefore, need not relate to a unique mechanism; conversely, different mechanisms may generate a common pattern.

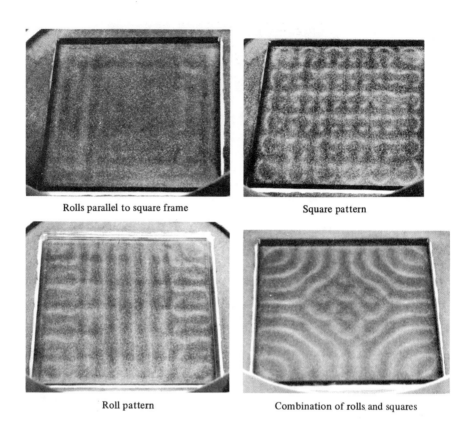

Rolls parallel to square frame

Square pattern

Roll pattern

Combination of rolls and squares

Figure 2. Layer of silicone oil being heated on a 12 cm² copper plate at a rate above threshold for dynamic pattern to form. [Koschmieder, 1966]

Buoyancy-driven convection patterns arise with a certain natural wavelength. If the boundaries intrude on the natural size, there is an obvious effect of the boundary on the pattern. Figure 2 shows a square dish in which the natural cell size is one-sixth or one-eighth the width of the dish. The boundaries impose a square pattern, whereas in the absence of boundaries there would be a hexagonal one.

If one heats the liquid more rapidly, i.e., beyond the threshold of instability, the pattern loses its regularity. Convection cells link up to form "vermicelli" or "roll cells," as they are referred to in hydrodynamics. If one "excites" the system by heating it still more strongly, other modes come into play (Whitehead, 1971). Figure 3, A and B, demonstrates an established cellular flow pattern that is influenced by the emergence of a different type of dynamic structure (roll cells). The interactions contribute to the wide range of dynamic structures that have been observed in natural convection systems (Whitehead, 1971).

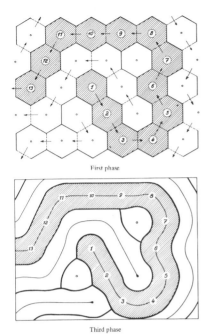

First phase

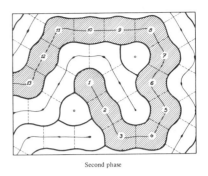

Second phase

Third phase

Figure 3. A. Diagrams based on experiments with layers of air laden with tabacco smoke. [Avsec, 1939]

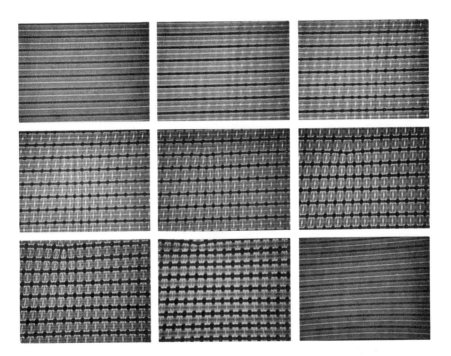

Figure 3. B. Layer of silicone oil being heated at about 12 times the rate shown in Figure 2 develops a three-dimensional dynamic pattern called bimodal convection. [Busse and Whitehead, 1971]

15

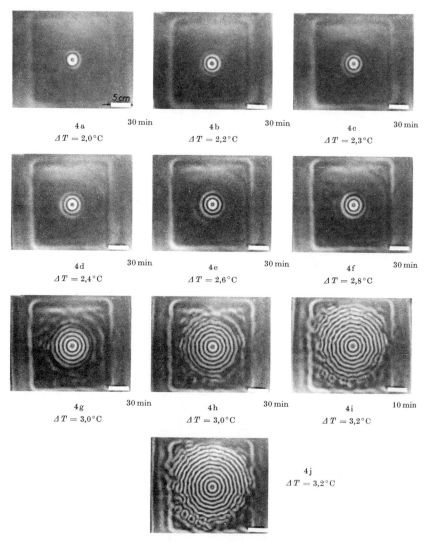

Figure 4. Layer of paraffin oil being heated on a flat plate, with additional local heating at the center. [Von Tippelskirch, 1959]

Figure 4 shows the effects of a local hot spot applied to a system that is close to its threshold of instability. This perturbation imposes a circular symmetry that loses its influence as it propagates outwards. At the corners, some of the "older" patterns can still be seen. Thus, interactions with the surround influence those patterns that would otherwise develop in a uniform system. Figure 5 shows a micrograph of a polymer film used to manufacture Baggies. A dynamic

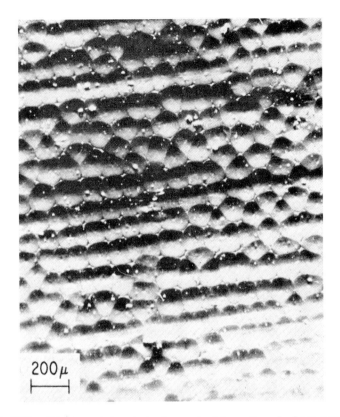

200μ

Figure 5. Diffuse light transmission photomicrograph of the surface of a Saran coating about 25 μ thick, deposited from mixed solvent. [Anand and Balwinski, 1969]

pattern is formed by the surface tension mechanism and set by the solvent evaporating from the surface (cf. Herbert Spencer's observation above). There may be an analog here to the prepattern concept in morphogenesis: biological structures may be "frozen in" from the original dynamic pattern; i.e., the permanent structure becomes a static record of the original dynamic pattern.

The electron micrograph (Figure 6) of Bangham and Horne (1962) shows a negatively stained preparation of cholesterol after treatment with saponin. The center-to-center spacing of the lattice is about 140 A, and the hole openings are about 80 A in diameter. Both values are in good agreement with those found for cell membranes treated with saponin by Dourmashkin and his co-workers (1962). Schulman and Rideal (1937) showed that saponin from an aqueous phase could penetrate into and complex with a number of surface-adsorbed lipids, particularly cholesterol, to form very insoluble

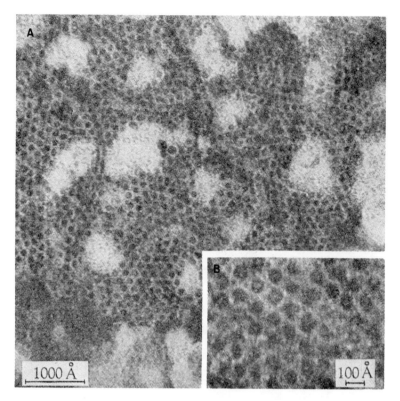

Figure 6. Electron micrograph of a negatively stained preparation of cholesterol after treatment with saponin. A. A region at low magnification showing the network interspersed with unreacted material. ×160,000. B. An area at higher magnification showing the hexagonal packing of "rings." ×500,000. [Bangham and Horne, 1962]

complexes. Thus, the hexagonal pattern here is the record of the dynamic pattern of diffusion, reaction, and precipitation during the saponin treatment, which also included staining.* The cholesterol

*It is not entirely self-evident that the cholesterol-saponin system is a manifestation of a dynamic pattern. Luzzati and Husson (1962) obtained hexagonal patterns from binary mixtures of soap and water and from multicomponent mixtures of brain lipids. The patterns are formed in a transitional phase between a crystalline solid (coagel) and a laminar structure of a liquid crystal. Those patterns are therefore explained on the basis of pure equilibrium considerations. The existence of the hexagonal phase has been confirmed by Stoeckenius (1962) by electron microscopy in identical material but fixed with osmium. Glauert and his co-workers (1962) present a model for the cholesterol-saponin system based on 20 associated subunits of 30-50 A wide cholesterol-saponin hydrophobic head groups arranged in a micell with the hydrophilic saponin sugar groups on the inside giving rise to the dark color in negative staining. With that model they obtain the 80 A diameter holes and 140 A center-to-center spacing. The presence of diffusion and complex formation is not a sufficient condition for the formation of dynamic patterns, because those processes can even take place in crystal formation and virus capsid self-aggregation. If the cholesterol-saponin system turns out to be a dynamic pattern it is one in Scriven's sense of the term (see page 12).

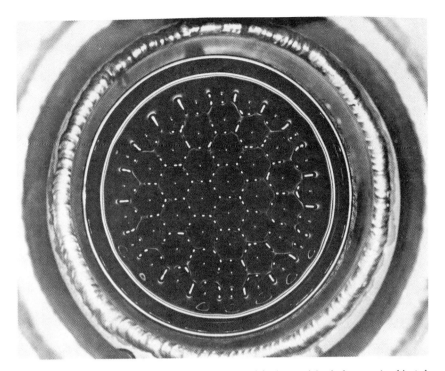

Figure 7. Layer of ferromagnetic liquid (suspension of ferrite particles in kerosene) subjected to a magnetic field slightly above threshold strength for configurational instability. The more isolated highlights represent peaks of the surface. [Cowley and Rosensweig, 1967]

solution was first dried on a carbon-coated cellulose grid. A drop of aqueous solution of 1% sodium phosphotungstate containing 0.005% white saponin was then placed on the grid; after 30 sec the drop was drained away and the grid examined in the electron microscope. Note that the pattern size is submicroscopic in this reaction-diffusion-precipitation system, the only one so far reported that displays hexagonal patterns (contrast this with the Liesegang rings discussed on page 30).

Figure 7 shows a pool of ferromagnetic liquid on which a perpendicular magnetic field is imposed. The surface has organized itself into a hexagonal tesselation with relief similar to that described in Figure 1. The dynamic processes pertain to electrical conduction and the maintenance of the magnetic field.

Dynamic patterns are also observed in geology, meteorology, and astrophysics. Figures 8 and 9 show dynamic patterns on a large scale in clouds and the solar coronasphere. Some meteorologists and astrophysicists believe that the pattern formation can be described in the same basic terms as the hydrodynamic patterns developed in

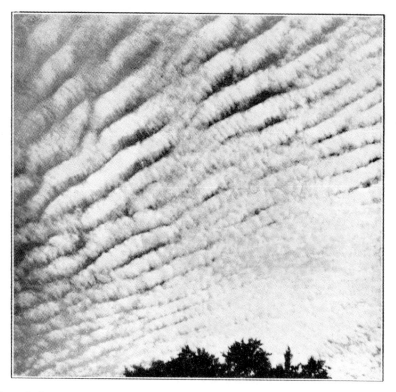

Figure 8. Photograph by C.P.J. Cave of roll-like cloud pattern, distinguished by "a curious series of cross bars developing across the main rolls." [Brunt, 1937]

laboratory experiments, although somewhat more complicated mechanisms are undoubtedly at work.

Figure 10 is an example of "patterned ground" in the arctic or high-altitude tundra. Alternate freezing and thawing cause large stones to migrate peripherally and fine material centrally to produce hexagonal patterns. Over many seasons the diurnal and seasonal temperature cycles can drive processes responsible for spatial structuring. The series of illustrations discussed above (Figures 1 to 10) show dynamic patterns with dimensions ranging from 10^{-6} to 10^6 meters, and the same principles obtain irrespective of the dimension of the system.

In elementary particle physics, Bohm (see Platt, 1970) identifies a "quantum jump" of an electron from one steady state of an atom to another as pattern restructuring. In his "process metaphysics," the steady-state patterns or "objects" can be understood only in a basic relationship to their environment with fields of flow extending

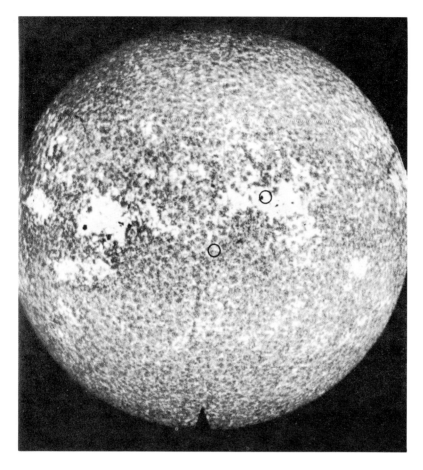

Figure 9. Calcium spectroheliogram taken on August 17, 1959, at Mount Wilson Observatory, showing solar granulation. Circle near the center indicates the nonmagnetic region; the other circle, the magnetic region. [Bahng and Schwarzschild, 1961]

outwards. Likewise, the environment takes on stable form, meaning, and points of reference only through the "objects" it sustains. Bohm also applies these ideas to electrons and other fundamental particles that are then assembled into larger but less stable patterns as in the following: atoms → living cells → organisms → brains → social networks → nations. The higher structures are built up in a "flow" hierarchy like a system of vortices. The structures are self-maintaining even though matter, energy, and information flow through them continually. (For similar ideas, see Anderson, 1972.)

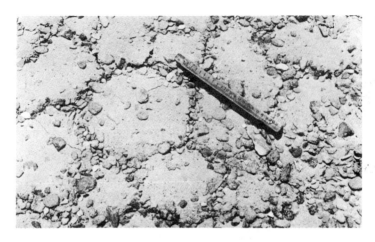

Figure 10. Photograph by A.E. Corte of sorted stone polygons. The ruler in the center is 23 cm long. [Washburn, 1956]

Examples of Mathematical Analysis of
Dynamic Systems

The branch of mathematics that applies to dynamic systems is called dynamic system theory and has its origin in Newtonian mechanics. Generally, dynamic systems arise from mechanics, where the state variables defining the instantaneous states of the system are represented by particle displacements and their corresponding moments. Dynamic descriptions, however, need not be limited to inanimate systems. In a recent monograph, Rosen (1970) presented a dynamic system theory for biologists. An earlier example, drawn from population biology, is found in the work of Volterra (1931) and in the independent studies of Lotka (1920, 1924, 1956) and others.

The Lotka-Volterra Scheme: A. Katchalsky

Volterra carried out an ecological study of the time-dependent changes in the size of Adriatic fish populations. The set of dynamic variables that constitute an appropriate instantaneous description of the system consists of the population sizes of the prey and predator. In order to formulate the equations of motion, Volterra had to specify how the populations interact.

At any given time, the prey population (x) is produced at a rate proportional to its own size $(k_1 x)$; i.e., reproduction occurs at an exponential rate and constitutes an "autocatalytic" step. At the same time, however, the prey is consumed by the predator at a rate $(k_2 xy)$ proportional to the sizes of both the predator and prey populations. By the same token, the size of the predator population (y) will grow at a rate $(k_3 xy)$ proportional to the sizes of both populations and decay at a rate $(k_4 y)$ proportional only to the population of the predator.

The interaction of the number of predators (y) and prey (x) can then be described by the following system of equations:

$$\frac{dx}{dt} = k_1 x - k_2 xy \qquad (1)$$

$$\frac{dy}{dt} = k_3 xy - k_4 y$$

An analysis of the behavior of dynamic system equations is often carried out in a phase plane; i.e., time is eliminated in the equations and the phase trajectories of the state variables x and y are plotted. The phase plane corresponding to Equation 1 yields a family of closed curves, each member of which is determined by a given set of rate constants in Equation 1 (Figure 11).

Because of its simplicity and its remarkable properties, the Lotka-Volterra scheme has had a major influence on biological thought. Its properties will be referred to below in the discussions of chemical oscillations, biological clocks, and time-dependent properties of neural networks.

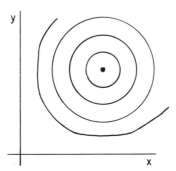

Figure 11. A phase plane diagram representing the trajectories of the Lotka-Volterra system. Each curve is determined by a given set of rate constants in Equation 1. [Blumenthal]

Relaxation Oscillators: Van der Pol's Equation: R. Blumenthal

Consider a particle with a single degree of freedom whose position is determined by a single displacement coordinate x. A one-dimensional harmonic oscillator is characterized by the particle's being subject to a single force whose magnitude is proportional to the displacement and whose direction is opposite to the direction of the displacement. If the mass of the particle is unity, Newton's second law reads

$$\frac{d^2 x}{dt^2} = -kx, \ k > 0 \tag{2}$$

where k is the "stiffness" of the oscillator and t is time.

The damped harmonic oscillator is characterized by the imposition of a further restoring force proportional to the velocity of the displaced particle. The faster the displaced particle is moving, the greater the new restoring force will be. According to Newton's second law,

$$\frac{d^2 x}{dt^2} = -kx - \beta\frac{dx}{dt} \tag{3}$$

where β, the new proportionality constant, is the viscosity. Plotting x versus t gives a damped oscillation.

The coefficient β, which measures the degree of damping of the system, is an interesting parameter. If we make β a given function of time, we may impose a force on the system. Furthermore, if β becomes a function of one of the state variables, the system develops a feedback loop. By choosing the following relation for β:

$$\beta(t) = -\epsilon(1 - x^2) \tag{4}$$

where ϵ is a small positive number, Equation 3 is converted to an equation for a relaxation oscillator—the well-known Van der Pol equation. The oscillation arises from a single closed trajectory called a *limit cycle*. Van der Pol (1922) established the equation in connection with vacuum tube amplifiers, but relaxation oscillators have been proposed as models for a wide variety of other physical and biological systems like the beating of the heart (Van der Pol and Van der Mark, 1928) and the nerve action potential (FitzHugh, 1969).

Chemodiffusional Systems: A. Katchalsky

From Aristotle on, the question of morphogenesis—the process by which biological form and pattern are generated—has challenged the natural philosopher. How does an initially homogeneous aggregate of cells develop differentiated characteristics? A possible answer is that the initially nonequilibrium but homogeneous state will be moved by random fluctuations towards a well-defined stable state. This idea was originally articulated by Rashevsky (1938) and again by Turing* (1952) in a paper titled "The Chemical Basis of Morphogenesis." Rashevsky based his development on a rather complex theory of diffusion-drag forces, whereas Turing had a more straightforward dynamic theory described as follows: An array of identical intercommunicating cells containing a number of identical chemical species called "morphogens" can undergo chemical reaction and diffusion. Initially, in an equilibrium and nonpatterned situation, the morphogens are distributed homogeneously over the cells. How can this system become unstable and then form a stable pattern? Turing illustrated a case of symmetry breaking by which we understand the emergence of crude patterns in the form of maintained concentration differences in the cells (Figure 12).

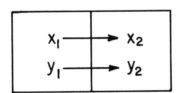

Figure 12. Two neighboring cells containing morphogens X and Y which can permeate between the cells. [Blumenthal]

Consider two cells, each containing two morphogens of concentrations x and y. The rate of reaction of x and y in either cell is given by

$$\left(\frac{dx}{dt}\right)_{\text{reaction}} = 5x - 6y + 1 \qquad (5)$$

$$\left(\frac{dy}{dt}\right)_{\text{reaction}} = 6x - 7y + 1$$

*This is the same man after whom the concept known as the "Turing machine" is named.

The rate of diffusion of x and y from cell 1 to cell 2 is given by

$$\left(\frac{dx}{dt}\right)_{diffusion} = 0.5(x_1 - x_2) \tag{6}$$

$$\left(\frac{dy}{dt}\right)_{diffusion} = 4.5(y_1 - y_2)$$

The numbers in Equations 1 and 2 for the reaction and diffusion rate constants are chosen for this special example. The total rate of change in cell 1 for x and y is

$$\frac{dx_1}{dt} = 5x_1 - 6y_1 + 1 - 0.5(x_1 - x_2) \tag{7}$$

$$\frac{dy_1}{dt} = 6x_1 - 7y_1 + 1 - 4.5(y_1 - y_2)$$

By inspection of Equation 7, it is immediately clear that when $x_1 = x_2 = 1$ and $y_1 = y_2 = 1$, $dx/dt = 0$ and $dy/dt = 0$. Knowledge of the reaction scheme, which is of the type represented by Equation 9 (see below), reveals that the system is at steady state where free energy is dissipated, rather than at equilibrium where the dissipation function is zero. But is this steady state stable? Steady states are generally regarded as stable, and, indeed, in the linear range* of nonequilibrium thermodynamics, the principle of minimum dissipation ensures stability. For the above system, one can test the stability by applying a perturbation to the homogeneous solution, $x_1 = x_2 = y_1 = y_2 = 1$. If a small increase in x_1 and y_1 makes dx_1/dt and dy_1/dt negative, then the system will revert on its own to the initial value, and the steady state is stable. If, on the other hand, dx_1/dt and dy_1/dt become positive, the fluctuation will be amplified, and the system will not return to its initial state.

If we introduce the following perturbations in x and y, $x_1 = 1.06$, $x_2 = 0.94$, $y_1 = 1.02$, and $y_2 = 0.98$, then $dx_1/dt = 0.12$ and $dy_1/dt = 0.04$. Matter will accumulate in cell 1 and be depleted in cell 2, thus breaking the symmetry of the system and establishing an inhomogeneous distribution.

---

*Steady states having linear relations between flows and forces are commonly regarded as being "near equilibrium," whereas those having nonlinear relations are regarded as being "far from equilibrium."

Nonequilibrium Steady States and Nerve Membrane Biophysics: W. Rall

Because some Work Session participants had only recently discovered the importance of nonequilibrium steady states to biology, Rall drew attention to a 35-year-old paper by Burton (1939) titled "The Properties of the Steady State Compared to Those of Equilibrium as Shown in Characteristic Biological Behavior." Burton wrote this lucid paper just before World War II, during his postdoctoral fellowship at the Universtiy of Pennsylvania.* When graduate teaching of physiology and biophysics was resumed after World War II, the concepts and implications brought out in Burton's paper were given central emphasis. At the University of Chicago, a series of five important papers on the steady-state kinetics of some biological systems was published by Hearon (1949a,b; 1950a,b,c) in which many points raised by Burton in qualitative form were reexamined more rigorously.

With regard to nerve membrane biophysics, the important papers of Hodgkin and Katz (1949) and Hodgkin and Huxley (1952) established the experimental evidence and the conceptual basis for understanding nerve membrane phenomena. The resting membrane is in a nonequilibrium steady state that depends upon free energy consumption by the sodium pump. This steady state is dominated by a membrane permeability to K^+ ions that is high relative to Na^+ permeability. However, when Na^+ permeability is made high relative to K^+ permeability, the membrane shifts away from the resting steady state towards an excited steady state. On this basis, the nerve action potential can be understood qualitatively as follows: A sufficient (threshold) amount of membrane depolarization results in a large and rapid increase in Na^+ permeability, which causes the membrane potential to shift rapidly towards an excited steady state. Before an excited steady state is reached, additional permeability changes reverse the trend. Both a decrease of Na^+ permeability and an increase of K^+ permeability cause the membrane potential to shift rapidly towards values near the resting value. The Hodgkin-Huxley (1952) mathematical model makes all this very explicit in terms of sodium and potassium conductances of their membrane equivalent circuit.

FitzHugh (1961, 1969) has given a valuable perspective of mathematical models of nerve excitation by classifying variables that specify the state of the system. His Type 1 includes the *measurable*

---

*Included in Burton's paper are references to earlier papers by A.V. Hill, S. Hecht, N. Rashevsky, and T. Teorell.

variables, i.e., those most easily measured, namely, membrane current and potential. Type 2 specifies the *excitation variables,* i.e., those that provide negative slope resistance or switching to provide regenerative action. Type 3 indicates the *recovery variables* that react upon variables of Types 1 and 2 to quench excitability, bring about recovery, and end the impulse. Their relaxation times are significantly longer than those of Types 1 and 2. Type 4 specifies *adaptation variables* that decrease excitability with still longer relaxation times.

In the context of the Work Session, Rall briefly referred to a particular mathematical model used to generate action potentials needed in a computational reconstruction of field potentials in the olfactory bulb (Rall and Shepherd, 1968). This model contains the *excitation* variable, ϵ, and the *recovery* variable, $\mathcal{J}$. ϵ represents the dimensionless ratio, G_ϵ/G_r, of excitatory membrane conductance to resting membrane conductance; it can be thought of as roughly proportional to sodium conductance. The variable, $\mathcal{J}$, represents the dimensionless ratio, $G\mathcal{J}/G_r$, of inhibitory or quenching membrane conductance to resting membrane conductance; it can be thought of as roughly proportional to potassium conductance. The equations can be expressed (for space clamp with total current clamped to zero) as follows, where v represents a normalized (dimensionless) membrane potential and T (dimensionless) represents time.

$$\frac{dv}{dT} = -v + (1 - v)\epsilon - (v + 0.1)\mathcal{J} \tag{8}$$

$$\frac{d\epsilon}{dT} = k_1 v^2 + k_2 v^4 - k_3 \epsilon - k_4 \epsilon \mathcal{J}$$

$$\frac{d\mathcal{J}}{dT} = k_5 \epsilon + k_6 \epsilon \mathcal{J} - k_7 \mathcal{J}$$

Because there are only two auxiliary variables and especially because the coefficients, k_1 to k_7, are all constants (some of which can be set to zero except for optimal shaping), this model is significantly simpler than the Hodgkin-Huxley one. This model does not pretend to fit all the data considered by Hodgkin and Huxley; its purpose was to use a simpler means of generating (in the time domain) an ϵ peak with a delayed $\mathcal{J}$ peak that would resemble the g_{Na} peak with a delayed g_K peak of Hodgkin and Huxley (Figure 13). Rall commented that the early rise and fall of g_{Na} (or ϵ) coupled with the overlapping later rise

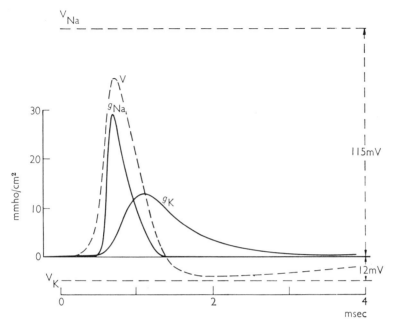

Figure 13. Theoretical solution for propagated action potential and conductances at 18.5°C. Total entry of Na⁺ = 4.33 pmole/cm² ; total exit of K⁺ = 4.26 pmole/cm² . g_{Na} and g_K = Na⁺ and K⁺ conductances; V_{Na} and V_K = Na⁺ and K⁺ equilibrium potentials; V = membrane potential. [Hodgkin and Huxley, 1952]

and fall of g_K (or $\mathscr{f}$) reminded him of the coupling between predator and prey populations studied by Lotka and Volterra. In particular, this similarity suggested a method of getting the rise of $\mathscr{f}$ (predator) to lag behind the rise of ϵ (prey) that is quite different from the procedure used by Hodgkin and Huxley to obtain a delayed rise of g_K. This approach has led to satisfactory action potentials, and fewer constant coefficients suffice to produce action potentials of less adjustable shape.

  More recently, Rall and Goldstein* have examined this mathematical model in terms of the phase plane plots and stability considerations previously described by FitzHugh (1961, 1969). When $\mathscr{f}$ is held constant, the reduced system (ϵ vs v) closely resembles FitzHugh's reduced Hodgkin-Huxley system obtained when n and h are held constant; the two isoclines intersect in three singular points (i.e., steady states where $d\epsilon/dT = 0 = dv/dT$). The outer two points represent

*W. Rall and S. Goldstein, unpublished calculations.

stable states (one resting and one excited) and the intermediate locus is a saddle point representing an all-or-none threshold property. However, when the Type 3 variables ($\mathscr{J}$, or n and h) are unlocked, interesting differences are revealed. Then, according to FitzHugh, the (unlocked) Hodgkin-Huxley model has neither a saddle point nor an excited state singularity, but only the resting state singularity. Rall and Goldstein found that their unlocked system retains three singular points (i.e., steady states where $d\mathscr{J}/dT = d\epsilon/dT = dv/dT = 0$), where the intermediate one is still a saddle point, and the excited state singularity has become a spiral instability. Further studies are in progress, and applications to action potential propagation in branching systems are being explored.*

Dynamic Patterns in Chemistry: A. Katchalsky, L. E. Scriven, and R. Blumenthal

Turing's equations (Equations 5 to 7) carry the prediction that a system of chemical reactions and diffusion may develop a dynamically maintained temporal and/or spatial pattern from an initially steady-state homogeneous distribution of matter. A spatial pattern in a pure chemical system was constructed by Liesegang (1906) who added a solution of NaCl and $AgNO_3$ on either side of a gel and observed the precipitation of AgCl in a regular pattern, the so-called Liesegang rings. This structure is, however, static and is based on a supersaturation phenomenon.

The occurrence of *temporal* patterns in chemical reaction systems has been known for decades (see review by Degn, 1972). Belousov (1958) continuously stirred potassium bromate, ceric sulfate, and citric acid in dilute sulfuric acid and found that the ratio of concentrations of the ceric (yellow) and cerous (colorless) ions oscillates, i.e., produces a recurring temporal pattern. In still another experiment, Zhabotinsky (1967) substituted malonic acid or other analogs for citric acid and could still obtain the oscillation (Figure 14).

---

*With regard to the participants' interest in theoretical dynamics of nervous systems, Rall pointed not only to the recent work of Wilson and Cowan (1972), but also to the earlier pioneering study of Householder and Landahl (1945) which has been included in Rashevsky's textbook (1948 edition). With regard to current interest in both stable and unstable steady states, transitions between such states, and hysteresis properties of possible biological importance, it is interesting to note that two chapters of Rashevsky's textbook (1938 and later editions) deal with hysteresis phenomena in physicochemical systems and in neural circuits.

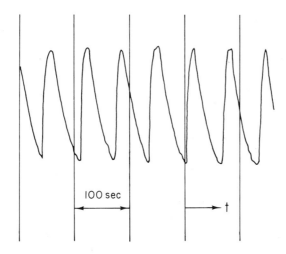

Figure 14. Oscillations of light absorption at 3650 A (filter UFS6) produced by the periodic change in Ce^{4+} ions. [Zhabotinsky, 1967]

Easily observable color changes may occur at a frequency of about 1 per min at room temperature.* The oscillation may be made even more visible by using a redox indicator such as ferrosin (a 0.01 M solution of 1-(ortho)phenanthroline ferrous sulfate is blue in an oxidizing solution and red in a reducing solution).

A remarkable *spatial* organization maintained by a dynamic system of chemical reactions is also well known. This is seen in the Belousov-Zhabotinsky systems. Busse (1969) reported that, if the Belousov reaction is not stirred and if the initial conditions are properly adjusted, the phenomenon of spatial patterning may be observed. Alternating stripes of oxidized and reduced forms of indicator appear and propagate through the solution, the mechanism being a system of coupled autocatalytic reactions.

Herschkowitz-Kaufman (1970) has studied further aspects of the spatial patterning of the Belousov-Zhabotinsky reaction. Starting with the theory of "dissipative structures" developed by Prigogine (1969; Prigogine et al., 1969), she has shown that the system, from initial instability, behaves in two ways. It develops a limit-cycle oscillation with respect to the concentrations of the constituents of the chemical reaction. The cycle has a defined period, a temporal pattern, that is independent of the initial perturbation. Secondly, a space-

*This reaction is excellently suited for classroom demonstrations (Field, 1972).

dependent perturbation will bring the system into a spatial organization called "dissipative structure" to contrast it from conventional structures found only in systems at thermodynamic equilibrium. As in the dynamics of neural populations, to be discussed below, a limit-cycle oscillation and a dissipative structure are interrelated, and Herschkowitz-Kaufman has demonstrated that link experimentally with the Belousov-Zhabotinsky reaction.

Whereas Busse (1969) had obtained the spatial organization by starting off with an externally imposed gradient, Herschkowitz-Kaufman (1970) showed that the spatial structure arose from a homogeneous system. The process is as follows: the reaction mixture is put into a test tube at constant temperature (21°C) and the stirring is discontinued. The solution starts changing color periodically from red to blue. The period depends on the initial concentration and temperature but is usually about 4 min. The oscillations start at a certain point and propagate in all directions at various speeds until a small concentric inhomogeneity appears, followed by the formation of alternate red and blue layers. The oscillations also continue in the part of the solution where structure has not been established. The space structure seems to result from an instability in the limit cycle itself. Lefelhocz (1972) has shown that the period of the limit cycle depends on the concentration of one of the chemicals and the temperature of the system.

Zaikin and Zhabotinsky (1970; Figure 15A) reported the spontaneous appearance in a free medium (having initially homogeneously distributed reactants) of a spatially periodic structure with a geometry different from that observed by Busse and Herschkowitz-Kaufman. Their reaction has been slightly modified by Winfree (1972) who placed the Belousov-Zhabotinsky reagents in a petri dish and added 1 g/l of Triton X-100 surfactant to facilitate spreading. As in the test tube, the reaction oscillates with a period of several minutes, turning from red to blue. Phase gradients in bulk oscillation, called "pseudo-waves" by Winfree, sweep across the reagent at variable speeds. One also observes the propagation of blue waves in concentric rings at a fixed velocity from certain points (Winfree's "pacemaker centers") with a temporal period shorter than that of the bulk oscillation. Unlike pseudo-waves, these waves, which propagate about 6 mm/min, are not reflected by the boundary of the dish, but are annihilated in head-on collisions with one another. By briefly tilting the dish, Winfree induced *spiral waves* that were first

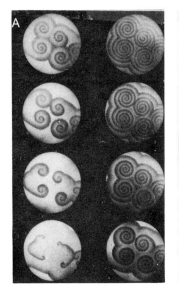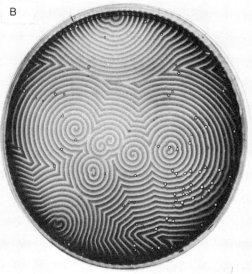

Figure 15. Spiral waves generated in a petri dish using the Belousov-Zhabotinsky reagents. A. Photograph of waves developing at different time intervals [Zhabotinsky]. B. Involute spiral waves propagating after disruption of spontaneously formed circular waves in a layer 1 mm in depth. Small circles are CO_2 bubbles. [Winfree, 1972]

described by Zhabotinsky (Figure 15B). Winfree (1972) recorded his observations as follows:

> An elaborate morphogenesis ensues in which segments of blue waves vanish. Near each free end is a center around which the remaining blue half-line propagates, winding into a spiral, as in the development of crystal growth spirals from a screw dislocation's line of emergence.

Since the Work Session, there has been increased activity and controversy in understanding the Belousov-Zhabotinsky reaction.* Two recent communications represent different schools of thought: the "reaction-diffusion" observed by DeSimone and his co-workers (1973) and the "local oscillator" seen by Kopell and Howard (1973). DeSimone and his collaborators (1973) carried out the reaction in cast membranes of hydrated collodion matrix containing substantial amounts of ferroin. In contrast to Winfree, these investigators found

*Papers were presented by A. Winfree and L.E. Scriven at the Aharon Katchalsky Memorial Symposium, Berkeley, California, 1973.

that hydrodynamic flows play no role in spiral wave initiation and that there is no evidence for pacemaker centers since new wave patterns appear randomly after washing the membranes. The role of diffusion was demonstrated by introducing slits in the membrane containing all the reagents, except ferroin, which is "membrane bound." For sufficiently narrow slits, communication by diffusion across a slit was effective.

The dynamic state of a developing pattern can be halted and recorded permanently by using membranes precoated with silver bromide. As dynamic patterns develop, the areas occupied by oxidized ferroin blacken with precipitate. The membranes can be washed and the state of the pattern at the time of washing recorded, thus providing a beautiful illustration of the prepattern concept.

Kopell and Howard (1973), on the other hand, observed formation and propagation of spatial patterns in the presence of an initial gradient in temperature or concentration of one or more reactants. According to these researchers, the bands form and propagate for strictly kinematic reasons, i.e., the oscillations occurring at different places in the fluid are independent of one another. Because the frequency of oscillation depends on the concentration of one of the reactants (Lefelhocz, 1972), the imposed concentration gradient provides a variation in frequency of the independent oscillators based on their location in the system. The macroscopic spatial patterns arise, therefore, from variations in frequency at different loci. Thus, Koppel and Howard conclude that diffusion is of negligible importance in the formation of bands.

In this section we dealt with the Belousov-Zhabotinsky reaction as an example of morphogenesis brought about by a nonlinear chemodiffusional system. Another aspect of dynamic chemical patterns is chemical wave propagation. The best-known examples are the burning of a fuse, the activation of a passive iron wire in concentrated nitric acid by the touch of a piece of zinc (Bonhoeffer, 1948, 1953), and the transmission of a nerve impulse in an axon. The analogies between the latter phenomena have been extensivley discussed by Bonhoeffer (1953). Originally, the system is at rest; however, after a perturbation of the system above a threshold value, the activation is not confined to the local perturbation but spreads out over the whole system as a chemical wave. (See page 27 for Rall's discussion on nerve conduction.)

Biological Systems

Turing's Theory of Morphogenesis: A. Katchalsky

Although a brief outline of the Turing model for morphogenesis has been presented above, a recapitulation of Turing's (1952) thoughts is best expressed in his own words:

> It is suggested that a system of chemical substances, called morphogens, reacting together and diffusing through a tissue is adequate to account for the main phenomena of morphogenesis. Such a system, although it may originally be quite homogeneous, may later develop a pattern or structure due to an instability of the homogeneous equilibrium, which is triggered off by random disturbances.

For mathematical convenience, although unrealistic biologically, Turing considered an isolated ring of cells in some detail. The morphogens X and Y are essentially metabolites in a morphogenetic process; a third substance (or class of substances), C, which is an evocator or catalyst in nature, is also involved. It is necessary to assume that X and Y diffuse at different rates and that a number of reactions involve X, Y, and the catalyst, C. These reactions do not merely use up the substances X and Y but also tend to produce them from other metabolites ("fuel substances") assumed to be abundantly present in the growing region; i.e., the morphogens are autocatalytic.

Initially, both X and Y are uniformly distributed, apart from chance fluctuations. The concentrations of X and Y will vary slowly as the system adjusts itself to a changing evocator concentration. Eventually, a point is reached where the system is unstable; the fluctuations, because they are no longer reversed, become cumulative. At this stage, the morphogen concentrations form a more or less regular wave pattern (Figure 16).

The progressive deepening of the waves will come to a stop when the concentration of one morphogen becomes almost zero. The cells that have accumulated morphogen will differentiate, whereas those that have extruded the morphogen will remain as they are. The pattern will regularize itself into a stationary wave that is almost perfectly symmetrical. Such a stationary wave, in a biological situation, might take the form of one of the morphogens accumulating in several cells,

36

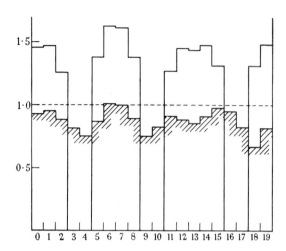

Figure 16. Development of concentration patterns of a morphogen (ordinate) in twenty linearly arranged cells (abscissa) of an organism. Dashed line = original homogeneous equilibrium; slant line = incipient pattern; solid line = final equilibrium. [Turing, 1952]

e.g., three, four, or more evenly distributed loci ("lobes") on a one-dimensional system such as the circumference of a circle. In an embryonic tissue, a regularly patterned distribution of metabolites may result ("prepatterning"), providing the basis for the inception of a morphological or histological pattern.

Turing's idealized model of the embryo may take two different forms. In one of them, the cell theory is recognized, but the cells are idealized geometric points (a discontinuous system). In the other, the matter of the organism is distributed continuously. The former situation could be applied to morphogenesis in hydra, where the number of tentacles that grow from a sphere is proportional to the surface area. Turing's mechanism could account for a regular variation in the distribution of morphogens on the surface of the sphere and the determination of the loci from which the tentacles would sprout. Other morphogenetic processes considered by Turing included whorled leaves, gastrulation, dappled patterns on skin, and phyllotaxis.

Analysis of Pattern and Rhythm: L. E. Scriven

Turing's work was significantly advanced by use of modern developments in systems analysis in a paper by Gmitro and Scriven (1966) entitled "A Physicochemical Basis for Pattern and Rhythm." These authors formulated mathematically the analysis of pattern and

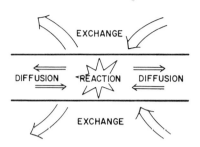

Figure 17. Diagram of basic system. Reaction and diffusion take place within or on a membrane or thread. There is also exchange with the surrounding media. [Gmitro and Scriven, 1966]

rhythm in surfaces or membranes and lines or fibers. In the basic system (diagrammed in Figure 17), within or on a membrane or thread that is uniform across its thickness, various chemical species react and diffuse along its length. At the same time, some, or all, of the participating species exchange with the surrounding media, and, at every location within the system, every chemical species obeys the conservation equation. The system can be expressed in the following terms:

Rate of accumulation within the system	=	Net rate of production by chemical reaction	+	Net rate of influx by diffusion along the system	+	Net rate of input by exchange with the surroundings

Gmitro and Scriven introduced the constitutive relations specifying the respective rate processes and then carried out the process of linearization by expansion of these rates in the Taylor series around the singular points: the uniform local steady-state concentration of the chemical species. They arrived at a linearized equation for small excursions from steady-state concentrations:

$$\frac{\partial x}{\partial t} = Kx + D\nabla^2 x \qquad (9)$$

where K and D are matrices and x is a column vector comprising the perturbations of the concentrations of chemical species from their steady-state values. In matrix K the Taylor coefficients for chemical reaction and exchange with the environment are lumped together, whereas D contains all the diffusional coefficients. Equation 9 is then solved by harmonic analysis of Fourier: any spatial pattern may be expressed as a weighted sum of members of a suitably chosen set of elementary patterns.

By choosing suitable pattern functions that are mathematically a complete set of eigenfunctions appropriate to the geometric configuration of the system of interest, Gmitro and Scriven (1966) were able to extend Turing's analysis of the origin of patterns in a ring of cells to a whole gamut of line-like and surface-like configurations.

A few of the findings of Gmitro and Scriven, which reinforce the indications that Turing had well in hand in the early 1950's, can be summarized as follows: Any uniform system of chemical reaction and diffusion suffers low-level noise that either comes from the surroundings or arises internally from molecular fluctuations. These disturbances may be either without effect or trigger the development of pattern and rhythm, according to the nature of sets of coefficients characterizing the reaction, exchange, and diffusion. In a system that is initially stable, a change in one of the reaction rates, as by enzyme activation, or in mobility of one of the constituents, may provoke instability in the system. There may be stationary patterns that grow in space, or propagating waves, or steady oscillations with different phases of different loci. When going from one to two, or to three or more participating chemical species, one finds that the range of possibilities becomes richer with each additional compound, leading to the emergence of entirely new behaviors. This property is of great interest to theoretically oriented developmental biologists.

Othmer and Scriven (1971) have applied some of these concepts to cellular network systems, emphasizing how instability and pattern formation are influenced by the preexisting pattern. With an eye towards developmental biology, they chose for a preexisting pattern various regular compartmentalizations of a system into discrete cells, each interchanging material with its nearest neighbors and with the surrounding bath of intercellular fluid. Thus, in passing from unicellular to multicellular systems, one encounters a new level of organization and complexity, a level stemming directly from cell-to-cell interactions of various types. Through chemical contact, cells may interchange one or more of their constituents, thereby altering metabolic states. In other words, chemical transformations taking place within individual cells may be influenced by mass transport between cells, and thereby differences in cell composition may be established. Inherent in this type of dynamic interaction are natural instabilities that may lead to spatial organization and temporal oscillations within groups of cells—the genesis of form and rhythm. Othmer and Scriven focused on these possibilities, taking chemical interactions for the model, even though there are, of course, other modes of intercellular communication.

Turing's original model was unquestionably overidealized, but it illustrated a principle that may be at work in reality. His isolated ring of cells, a matter of convenience for conceptualization, may seem to be a "spherical horse" to those who have difficulty grasping the principle and its implications.* Othmer and Scriven analyzed geometries that are somewhat more complex than Turing's model. Their results show that the dynamic pattern is strongly influenced by the way in which the network of cells is hooked up, i.e., the topology or connectivity of the network, or, from another point of view, the preexisting pattern. Changes in permeability between two cells can transform the entire network from a stable to an unstable system. This illustrates one way in which the collective behavior can be controlled locally by junctional transport. Local control can also be exerted through boundary conditions that represent interaction of the system with its environment or with an internal source. The results indicate that chemical signals can be propagated as concentration waves traveling at speeds some magnitudes greater than those allowed by diffusion.

Dissipative Structures: A. Katchalsky

Prigogine, Nicolis, Lefever, and their co-workers in Brussels have taken up Turing's considerations on stability, structure, and fluctuations from slightly different vantage points. They have modified and extensively investigated the properties of one of the reaction schemes that, according to Turing, gives rise to instability and structuring:

$$A \overset{k_1}{\to} X \tag{10a}$$

$$2X + Y \overset{k_2}{\to} 3X \tag{10b}$$

$$B + X \overset{k_3}{\to} Y + D \tag{10c}$$

$$X \overset{k_4}{\to} E \tag{10d}$$

$$\overline{A + B \to E + D} \tag{10e}$$

*During this discussion at the Work Session, Katchalsky told one of his famous stories: A rich man, interested in breeding race horses, commissioned three experts, a veterinarian, a mechanical engineer, and a theoretical physicist, to find out the best properties of race horses. After a year, the experts reported the results of their investigation: the veterinarian had undertaken a genetic study and concluded that brown horses are the fastest, and the engineer came to the conclusion that thin legs give optimal qualities for racing. The theoretical physicist did not give up his quest at the end of one year; he merely asked for more time to study the question, claiming progress in solving the case of the spherical horse.

where A, B, E, and D are the initial and final products and X and Y are the independent variables. The autocatalytic step (Equation 10b) involves a trimolecular reaction. Setting the k's equal to unity, the following kinetic equations are obtained:

$$\frac{dX}{dt} = A + X^2Y - BX - X \qquad (11)$$

$$\frac{dY}{dt} = BX - X^2Y$$

Based on a stability analysis, this system of equations becomes unstable when $B > B_c$, where B_c is a critical value for the concentration of substance B and $B_c = 1 + A$. The onset of this instability is arrived at by varying B while maintaining A constant. Lefever and Nicolis (1971) have shown that this set of reactions will exhibit limit-cycle oscillatory behavior beyond that unstable point.

     Figure 18 shows a phase plane representation of the limit cycle for a variety of different initial conditions. Lefever and Nicolis (1971) proved that the limit cycle is unique and stable with respect to small fluctuations. Furthermore, they consider the marginal stability as corresponding to a "bifurcation point" where the stable focus either develops into a stable limit cycle or into an unstable focus.

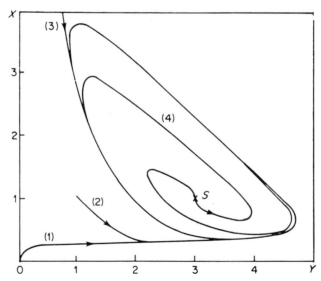

Figure 18. Trajectories obtained by numerical integration of Equation 11 for (1) $X = Y = 0$; (2) $X = Y = 1$; (3) $X = 10$, $Y = 0$; (4) $X = 1$, $Y = 3$. S = steady state. [Lefever and Nicolis, 1971]

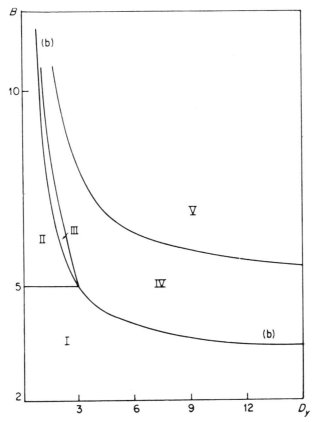

Figure 19. Stability regions and steady states as a function of B (see the text) and the diffusion coefficient, D_Y, of species Y. In domain I only the stable homogeneous steady state exists. In regions II, III, and V no time-independent stable state exists, whereas in region IV the inhomogeneous steady state is stable. [Lefever, 1968]

The appearance of a chemical "dissipative structure" is demonstrated in the following way: Consider the reaction shown in Equation 11 as if it were going on in two boxes and that X and Y diffuse between the boxes at different rates. The critical value for B is dependent on the diffusion coefficients of X and Y. For constant A at that critical value of reactant B, the concentrations of X and Y in compartments 1 and 2 begin to differ. As shown in Figure 19, there is a range of B concentrations in which the *inhomogeneous* solution is stationary.

Generalizing this two-component analysis, Lefever (1968) calculated the stable distribution of matter in a 50-cell system for the reaction given by Equation 10. His results are shown in Figure 20.

42

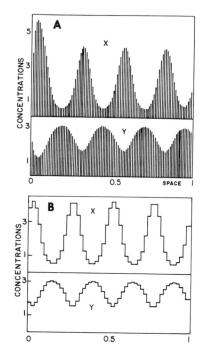

Figure 20. A. Steady state distributions for a series of 100 boxes with fixed concentrations $X = 2$ and $Y = 2.62$ at the boundaries. B. Steady state distributions for a series of 50 boxes with periodic boundary conditions; same numerical values as in A. [Lefever, 1968]

For many years, Prigogine and his collaborators in Brussels have attempted to extend the concepts of nonequilibrium thermodynamics into the nonlinear range. They have been searching for a general minimal evolutionary principle in order to devise a means to predict the fate of a system. So far, they have furnished only a partial answer in terms of a "thermodynamic" stability criterion. A summary of their endeavor, stated in terms of dissipative function and steady states, has been reported by Katchalsky (1971) and is known as the "Glansdorff-Prigogine stability criterion." However, Glansdorff and Prigogine refer to it as "excess entropy production."*

The Phase-Shift Model

Goodwin and Cohen (1969), believing that the Turing model would not hold up against the problems of regulation, regeneration, the

*Recently, Glansdorff and his collaborators (1974) summarized the formulation of their stability criterion in response to qualms expressed by Keizer and Fox (1974) regarding the range of validity of the Glansdorff-Prigogine criterion of stability of nonequilibrium states.

time required to establish a standing wave, and stability in the presence of cell movement, have provided an alternative model. They regard development as the result of a well-defined sequence of events in which spatial and temporal organizations in the developing tissue are ultimately connected. Prior to any visible sign of spatial organization, they propose that there must be a specific distribution of differing cell *states,* a state being defined as the amplitude and period of a limit cycle in a cell in which a multitude of chemical species are involved (see the discussion on macrostates on page 94). Localized clocks or pacemakers are postulated to send out "organizing waves" of activity in the developing tissue. By functional coupling, the cells are entrained by the fastest cell in the pacemaker region.

This may be visualized in the following way. Within each cell, an autonomous periodic event, S (for synchronizing the organizing property of the event), occurs that involves an assembly of different biochemical species. A signal that can be transmitted by small ions or molecules is transmitted to neighboring cells and induces an S event therein and in other places. Forward propagation, and thereby polarity, is guaranteed by assuming a refractory period following the signaling during which S cannot be induced. The polarity then establishes an embryonic axis in relation to which positional information may be measured. Other pacemakers also send out organizing waves of the S event at different frequencies so that a "frequency gradient" will be established.

In order to obtain finer positional information within an "S region" or field, defined by Wolpert (1969) as "that region in which all cells having their positional information specified with respect to the same set of points," a second periodic event, P (for phase), is postulated. The P event is propagated from the origin at a definite phase angle with respect to the S event, but, because it is propagated more slowly, the phase angle increases with distances from the reference point. In that fashion, the temporal organization of an individual cell is converted by the functional coupling between cells into a *spatial ordering.*

Other developmental phenomena that the Goodwin-Cohen model has been invoked to explain include regeneration in *Hydra,* positional information in the amphibian embryo, retinal-tectal projection of the vertebrate visual system, and more recently, slime mold morphogenesis (see "Cell Patterning" below).

An Alternative View of Morphogenesis

Generally, it is very difficult to subject Turing's theory for the chemical basis of morphogenesis to an experimental test, because neither the morphogens nor their reaction rates and diffusion coefficients are known for any real organism. However, if one considers an organism whose development can be followed and manipulated experimentally, a number of experimental criteria can be set up, based on the developmental pattern, to test the validity of Turing's theory. Such an approach is presently being taken by Gordon and Drum.*

In the preceding sections, we have seen that the following factors are characteristic of the development of a dynamic pattern: (1) There should be uniformity of spacing, a condition that is necessary, but not sufficient, for a Turing mechanism. (2) In a short period after the onset of instability, there is no appearance of a major pattern which dominates. If one can freeze the pattern shortly after its main features are formed, one should see imperfections owing to the presence of a number of growing patterns. (3) There is a characteristic wavelength of the dominant pattern independent of the size or shape of the organism. It should be feasible to test this feature, e.g., the spacing of the stripes in zebras should be the same for the adult as well as for the young animal.

Gordon and Drum* set out to apply these criteria to morphogenesis of the diatom shell (*Navicula* and *Licomorpha*), an organism whose development may be manipulated experimentally. In addition to regularly spaced stripes, the photograph of the shell (Figure 21) shows many instances of branching that become very dramatic in mutant strains of *Licomorpha*. Although a Turing mechanism could, perhaps, account for the formation of stripes, it cannot explain the branching. (The Belousov-Zhabotinsky reaction shows no evidence of branching.) Gordon and Drum believe that nature may have chosen a simpler method, e.g., a frost-like precipitation of what could be a single substance (such as silica), which explains the regular pattern as well as the branching. They have thus been able to describe the development of a biological pattern that does not necessarily conform to, and part of which is still unexplained by, a Turing mechanism. Therefore, Turing's theory has, according to Gordon and Drum, failed to justify the claim of being "the chemical basis of morphogenesis."

*R. Gordon and R.W. Drum: "On diatom shell morphogenesis: a test of Turing's theory" (manuscript in preparation).

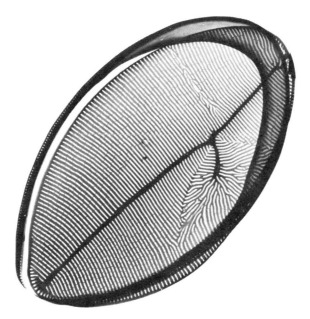

Figure 21. *Licomorpha* shell with branched "midrib." Note the branchings and terminations of the finer striae, explainable in terms of accretionary growth from the midrib. [Gordon and Drum]

Dissipative Peptide Synthesis: A. Katchalsky

In Katchalsky's laboratory, the polycondensation of amino acid adenylates in aqueous media was carried out for many years as a model system for prebiotic evolution. Only polypeptides with molecular weights too low to be considered serious candidates for prebiotic evolution of biopolymers were obtained. In 1951, Bernal suggested that formation of primitive biopolymers in a homogeneous aqueous medium, such as the ocean, is highly improbable because it would require a heterogeneous catalytic surface to accumulate monomers and protect them from hydrolysis. Katchalsky (see Paecht-Horowitz et al., 1970) followed this up by adding montmorillonite, a hydrated silicate of aluminum (one of the important clay minerals), to the reaction mixture. Whereas without the clay, the yield of polypeptides decreases monotonically with increasing molecular weight, with it, one obtains many compounds of higher molecular weight. When the yield of the synthesized polypeptide is plotted against its molecular weight (Figure 22), a definite band pattern is evident. The factor that controls the molecular weight pattern is nonlinear polymerization coupled with

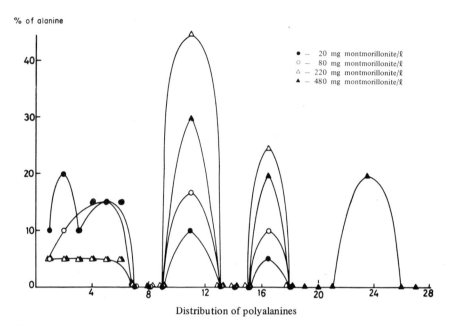

% of alanine

Figure 22. Distribution of the molecular weights of polyalanines, obtained when alanine adenylate is introduced into an aqueous solution at pH 8.5 in the presence of various amounts of montmorillonite. [Katchalsky, 1971]

lateral diffusion over a heterogeneous surface (the clay) which can accumulate precursors and protect them from hydrolysis. Katchalsky (1971) suggested that this is a dynamic pattern subject to the same principles of formation and maintenance as discussed above. Moreover, he emphasized the general utility of the dynamic pattern concept for understanding the genesis of early structures from which life arose.

Eigen's Theory of Self-Organization of Matter

Eigen's (1971a) theory of molecular self-organization and evolution relates closely to the concept of dynamic patterns discussed in the foregoing sections. The theory's thermodynamic foundations rely heavily on the concepts and criteria developed by Glansdorff and Prigogine (1971) whose work has led Eigen to draw the following conclusions: Selection and evolution cannot occur in systems at, or close to, equilibrium even if the right types of substances are present. Autocatalysis will not result in growth for near-equilibrium systems, because catalytic enhancement influences both forward and reverse reactions in the same way, and thus no source of free energy can be established to maintain the system far from equilibrium. Whereas Prigogine and others believe that dissipative spatial structures are important for the genesis of functional order in evolution, Eigen does not regard them as the key to understanding biological self-organization. The first steps may even have occurred in a structureless "soup," involving functional macromolecular structures such as nucleic acid and proteins. Eigen's theory leads to the emergence of functional order among a tremendously complex variety of chemical compounds, possibly in a homogeneous phase. The organization develops in an "information space" rather than in a geometric space. The use of the Glansdorff-Prigogine principle requires new variables such as "selection strains" and "selection values" to replace the convectional "forces" and "flows" in the thermodynamics of irreversible processes.

The process of molecular self-organization includes many random events that do not have any instructed functional significance. Eigen sorts out how certain random events are fed back to their origin and thereby become the cause of amplified action. Under certain external conditions, the multiple interplay between cause and effect will build up to a macroscopic, functional organization. The "value" concept forms the basis for a "new" information theory that includes the origin of self-organization of "valuable" information, thereby uniting Darwin's evolution principle with classical information theory.

Eigen has considered concrete reaction models, i.e., complementary instruction in nucleic acids and cyclic catalysis in an enzyme reaction sequence. From his results, he concludes that neither nucleic acids nor proteins *alone* can start any significant type of functional self-organization. Rather, a combination of the self-instructive property of complementary recognition (nucleic acids) *together with* the enormous functional capacity of proteins is required.

Eigen has also introduced the "hypercycle" (Figure 23), embodying a "cycle hierarchy," in which many cyclic complementary nucleotide collectives are linked together with an enzyme reaction cycle. The "hypercycle" has the following properties: (1) autocatalytic growth, (2) competition between cycles for selection, (3) sharp, possibly "all-or-none," selection at the singularities by nonlinearity, (4) utilization of small selective advantages (e.g., dominance of L - over D -amino acids in proteins), (5) large information capacity (optimized) with small individual sequences, (6) evolution, i.e., utilization of genotypic mutations in the cycles, (7) selection against parasitic branches, (8) matching of branching and cycle, (9) compartmentalization, and (10) individualizing of a system.

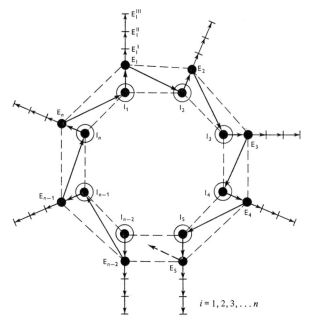

Figure 23. The self-instructive catalytic hypercycle. The I_i represent information carriers, i.e., complementary single strands of RNA. Each small cycle indicates the self-instructive property of the I_i collective involving the two complementary strands. The E_i (encoded by I_i) represent catalytic functions. Each branch may include several functions (e.g., polymerization, translation, control), one of which has to provide a coupling to the information carrier I_{i-1} (e.g., enhancement of the formation of I_{i+1} by specific recognition). The trace representing all couplings must close up, i.e., there must be an E_n which enhances the formation of I_1. The hypercycle is described by a system of nonlinear differential equations. [Eigen, 1971a]

All the features of dynamic flows underlying organization and hierarchical jumps to new levels are inherent in Eigen's theory. In fact, his theory provided a quantitative basis for the development of laboratory experiments in evolution by Spiegelman (1971) on the $Q\beta$ phage replicase system.

Eigen (1974) has also proffered the tantalizing possibility that these principles may be applied to self-organization in neural populations (e.g., memory), where the factors of internal redundancy, feedback, competition, and superimposed "value" are prevalent.

Cell Patterning

Cellular slime molds, *Dictyostelium discoideum,* are extensively utilized as models for developing systems. Their life cycle starts with the rupture of a spore and the emergence of amoebas that are motile and move over the surface of an agar-coated petri dish, feeding on bacteria by phagocytosis. After exhausting the food supply, the individual cells aggregate into a multicellular slug that is capable of independent movement. Eventually, the slug stops moving and develops into a multicellular fruiting body. When the amoebas that are capable of aggregating are uniformly plated on a surface, they will distribute themselves into a number of territories, and aggregation will proceed within each grouping.

It has been shown that slime mold amoebas are attracted chemotactically to a compound identified in *D. discoideum* as adenosine 3',5'-phosphate (cyclic AMP) that is synthesized by the cells during the period of aggregation. The same species has been found to produce phosphodiesterase, which converts cyclic AMP to chemotactically inactive 5'-AMP. This enzyme acts extracellularly.

Keller and Segel (1970) view initiation of slime mold aggregation as an onset of instability caused by changes in the basic parameters that characterize the system. These authors formulate the instability and subsequent pattern formation in the following way: the amoeba concentration is described by a continuous function $a(x,y,t)$ where x and y represent spatial coordinates and t, time. Similarly, $\rho(x,y,t)$ and $\eta(x,y,t)$ represent the local, time-dependent concentrations of cyclic AMP and phosphodiesterase, respectively. Equations for the rates of change were derived by taking into account the following basic processes: (1) production of cyclic AMP at a rate of $f(\rho)$ per amoeba, (2) production of phosphodiesterase at a rate of $g(\rho,\eta)$ per amoeba, (3) a Michaelis-Menten type of kinetics for the reaction between cyclic AMP and phosphodiesterase, (4) Fick's diffusion law for the chemical species, and (5) changes in amoeba concentration due to directional chemotactic movement towards a positive gradient of amoebas and to random motion analogous to diffusion.

Taking into account steady-state kinetics for the enzyme-substrate reaction, Keller and Segel reduced the system to two basic equations for the rates of change of cyclic AMP and concentration of amoebas, respectively:

$$\frac{\partial \rho}{\partial t} = -k(\rho)\rho + af(\rho) + D_\rho \nabla^2 \rho \tag{12}$$

$$\frac{\partial a}{\partial t} = - \nabla(D_1 \nabla \rho) + \nabla(D_2 \nabla a)$$

where $k(\rho)\rho$ indicates the chemical decay rate of cyclic AMP and includes the total concentration of enzyme, the decomposition rate of the substrate-enzyme complex, and the Michaelis-Menten constant for the complex. D_ρ and D_2 are the Fick diffusion constants for cyclic AMP and amoebas, respectively, whereas D_1 is a "chemotactic coefficient," indicating the influence of the cyclic AMP gradient on the flow of amoebas.

After going through the linearization and normal mode analysis, Keller and Segel arrived at equations for local disturbances of homogeneity at the marginal stable point:

$$\rho = \rho_0 + \epsilon D_2 \cos qx \exp (\sigma t) \tag{13}$$

$$a = a_0 + \epsilon D_1 \cos qx \exp (\sigma t)$$

where ϵ is a small parameter left indeterminate by linear analysis, and q is the wave number of the system (see Figure 24).

The theory predicts that at the onset of instability the cells should increase (1) their sensitivity to a given cyclic AMP gradient, (2) their rate of cyclic AMP production, or (3) the stimulation of cyclic AMP production by cyclic AMP. It has been shown that both sensitivity to cyclic AMP and its production rate rise 100-fold in *D. discoideum* during a period extending from the onset of aggregation (Shaffer, 1962; Bonner et al., 1969).

During cell aggregation, waves of fast inward movement (towards the group center) are often observed, possibly owing to a series of directional pulses paced by the center. Keller and Segel regard these as a manifestation of so-called overstability in which the breakup of equilibrium occurs in an oscillatory manner. Robertson and Cohen (1972), on the other hand, regard the pacemaking centers that send out organizing waves as the quintessence of slime mold morphogenesis and describe the event in the following way: The period of differentiation after exhaustion of the food supply is called interphase. Some cells begin to secrete almost periodic pulses of cyclic AMP lasting less than 2 sec for a period of approximately 5 min. The amplitude is reduced both by diffusion and by action of extracellular phosphodiesterase. When a suprathreshold concentration of cyclic AMP hits the sensitive region of the membranes of neighboring amoebas, these, in turn, will start pulsing. The signal and response mechanisms lead to an outwardly propagated wave of inward movement that is repeated periodically, and the cells tend to move in a stream joined towards the center.

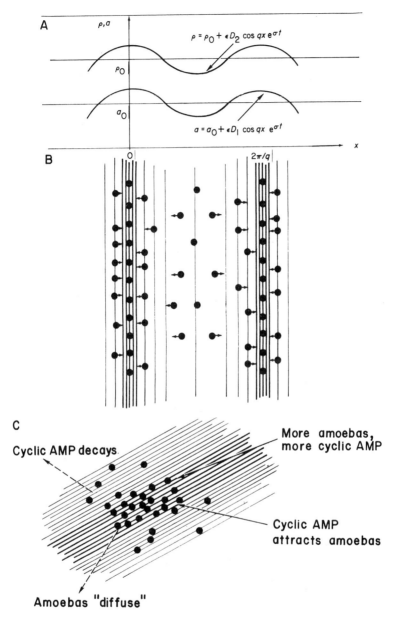

Figure 24. A. Graph showing sinusoidal perturbation of cyclic AMP density (a) and amoeba density (ρ). B. Corresponding "streaks" of relatively high amoeba (•) concentration and cyclic AMP (vertical lines) concentration. The arrows in this schematic diagram show the direction of amoeba motion. Superposition of "streaks" can give "clouds." C. Reaction to local concentration of amoebas (•) and cyclic AMP (slanted lines) when cyclic AMP production rate is constant. Solid arrows indicate tendencies to increase the local concentration still further. Dashed arrows indicate tendencies to return local concentration to equilibrium values. Instability occurs if the former tendency outweighs the latter. [Keller and Segel, 1970]

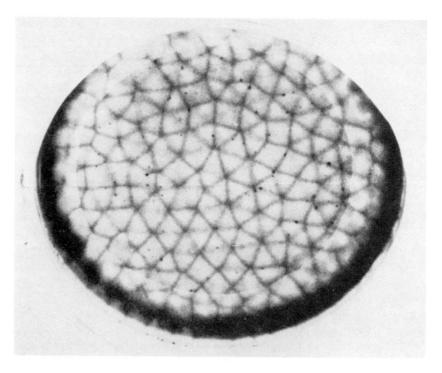

Figure 25. Pattern formed by actively motile *Euglena gracilis* var. *bacillaris* in an acid liquid medium in a petri dish 5 cm in diameter. Depth of liquid about 0.5 cm. [Robbins, 1952]

Robertson and Cohen (1972) corroborated their theory of slime mold development by performing a series of experiments in which they delivered pulses of cyclic AMP periodically to a field of amoebas during interphase by electrophoresis from a micropipette. The experiments demonstrated to their satisfaction that the nature and timing of the responses follow the general picture of organizing waves that control a developing field.

Dynamically patterned organization of unicellular organisms has been observed in *Euglena* (Figure 25) by Robbins (1952) and in *Tetrahymena* (Figure 26) by Hartman and High (1974). Figure 26 shows a fairly dense culture of *Tetrahymena* that has formed a pattern 12 sec after stirring. This is a particularly intriguing example of a dynamic pattern and invites analogy with either the buoyancy or the surface tension mechanisms discussed above (see page 13). The physical processes underlying *Tetrahymena* pattern formations have recently been analyzed by Hartman and High (1974).

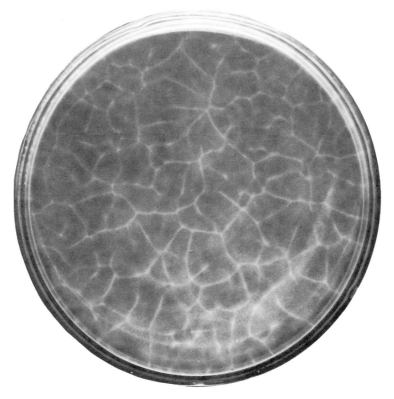

Figure 26. Two-dimensional bioconvection patterns in *Tetrahymena pyriformis*. The culture is in a dish 100 mm in diameter, and the fluid is 0.6 cm deep. [Hartman and High, 1974]

Terminology and Essential Features

Up to this point, we have discussed how the concept of dynamic patterns has developed in various disciplines, using the terminologies of the authors whose work was being described. For the Work Session, Katchalsky launched the term "cooperative nonequilibrium phenomena" as a leitmotiv. He used the term "cooperative" in the sense of classical physics in which the transition in system behavior from a single molecule to an assembly of molecules is described. The classical example is magnetization of an assembly of ferromagnites as described by the well-known Ising model (see Hill, 1967). The problems of cooperativity are not yet fully decided; e.g., the problem of a three-dimensional Ising model has not yet been solved. In statistical mechanics, the notion of cooperativity leads to an understanding of phase transitions from solid to liquid to vapor. As an example of "cooperative nonequilibrium phenomenon," Blumenthal and his co-workers (1970) analyzed a membranous structure that is built up of cooperative interacting elements exposed to nonequilibrium forces and flows such as diffusion (see pages 65 to 70). They found that transmembrane flow of material that interacts with the membrane elements undergoing a cooperative structural transition leads to a new hierarchy of organization.

At the Work Session, Katchalsky extended this concept to cooperativity based exclusively on the interaction of flows. These interactions generate dynamically maintained patterns (sometimes called "flow structures" or "dissipative structures" according to Prigogine).

Dynamic patterns or dissipative structures describe self-organization in space but need not be limited to that context. In his work on the theory of evolution (see pages 46 to 48), Eigen does not use the geometric aspect of self-organization in "information space." Similarly, in the study of neural populations, it is the information and not the geometric space that is given primary emphasis (see Chapter III).

An annoying ambiguity attaches to the word "structure." It traditionally refers to static *spatial* patterns that are near or at thermodynamic equilibrium. But the word has been extensively adopted in the temporal domain and in thermodynamics to apply to systems with recognizable patterns maintained for finite periods however brief or enduring. These patterns differ significantly, however, from the old space structure in their requirement of energy for their maintenance. Thus, the classical structure-function dichotomy in biology is blurred by the introduction of dissipative structure, or what is, in effect, a functional or dynamic structure as contrasted with the older static one. For these reasons, we adhere to the term dynamic patterns.

This proposed terminology may seem limited to the description of self-organization in Euclidean space. As may be noted from Eigen's work on the theory of evolution, the geometric aspect of self-organization is unimportant; the concept of dynamic patterns leads to self-organization in "information space." Similarly, in neural populations, it is not the geometric but the information space that must be considered.

Katchalsky emphasized three essentials for a system to exhibit dynamic patterns: (1) the system should have a sufficient density of interacting elements, (2) the interactions between the elements should be nonlinear, and (3) free energy should be dissipated by the system. Dynamic patterns can be established only in a region far from equilibrium, where the relations between forces and flows are highly nonlinear and jump transitions between steady states can occur. In dynamic patterns, the transitions can occur at more than one critical point, giving rise to a series of new spatial and temporal organizations of matter. Katchalsky termed such assemblies of multiple steady states as "a spectral hierarchy of dynamic patterns."

Scriven, on the other hand, listed the following as the key processes underlying the genesis of dynamic patterns: one or more transformation processes, one or more transport processes, and interference between the two types of processes. The last refers, for example, to diffusion interfering with the buildup of a local concentration of chemical species produced by chemical reaction and vice versa. Scriven pointed out that the requirement of dissipation (energy, etc.) is *not* an essential, inasmuch as standing waves and other dynamic patterns are commonplace in nondissipative systems.* In this regard, Scriven feels that there is a significant distinction between the concept of dynamic pattern and the notion of dissipative structure, the former including the latter and emphasizing the importance of interfering transport and transformation.

The Macrostate Concept

Goodwin (1963), whose monograph, "The Temporal Organization in Cells," provides a quantitative general theory of organization, shows that the state of an individual cell involves specification of the position-dependent concentrations of approximately 10^4 molecular species, intimately coupled by nonlinear laws of mass action (chemical reactions) along with inflow and outflow terms (diffusion). He introduced a statistical-mechanical analog in terms of cellular control processes to describe cell behavior and attempted to find for the cell state a correlate of the thermodynamic variables that describe the overall properties of a gas (e.g., temperature, entropy, and pressure). In

---

*The Liesegang rings (page 30) and Herbert Spencer's honeycomb structure (page 11) are considered by Scriven to be dynamic patterns, because they are generated by interfering processes of transformation and transport. Katchalsky, however, considered them to be "typical static structures" (verbatim quote from the transcript of his lecture on May 14, 1972, at the NRP), because no energy is required to maintain the structures. The opposing views of Scriven and Katchalsky are also evident in Figures 5, 6, and 10, which Scriven describes as examples of dynamic patterns, whereas Katchalsky would have considered them to be static structures.

considering a theoretical "macrostate" for a neural population, Cowan (1970) attempted to find a statistical-mechanical correlate to describe the macrostate in terms of the firing pattern of 10^9 neurons in a subpopulation (see Chapter III below).

Similarly, Kerner (1971) described large ecosystems where speciation is typically high (10^6 to 10^8 species "heavily weighted with beetles") using the Gibbs ensemble theory, the classic, statistical, thermodynamic treatment of ensembles of molecules in terms of a macrostate. The description applies an extension of the Lotka-Volterra ecodynamics to this large assembly of species (May, 1972).

Goodwin (1963) arrived at a description of complex biochemical interactions and metabolic pathways in terms of conservative oscillatory processes. In this manner, the state of a cell can be specified by the amplitude and phase of a cycle of a multiplicity of chemical species and their interactions. He introduced the term "talandic" (from the Greek, meaning oscillation) to emphasize the dynamic and oscillating character of all the variables measured in the investigation of epigenetic (developmental) phenomena. The theoretically derived quantities are thus termed talandic temperature, energy, and entropy, in analogy to the corresponding thermodynamic variables describing gases. The drawback of Goodwin's theory is that the statistical-mechanical treatment can only be applied to linear or nonlinear conservative oscillators, such as the Lotka-Volterra oscillation (see page 22). The only known biochemical oscillation, the glycolytic cycle (see page 60), obeys nonlinear dissipative dynamics, such as the Van der Pol or limit-cycle oscillation (see page 24). One of the essential differences between the two types of oscillations is that perturbations of the conservative oscillator will move it into another orbit or frequency, whereas the limit-cycle oscillator will maintain its orbit or frequency upon perturbation. It is likely that biochemical oscillators will be similar to the glycolytic cycle, because oscillators that cannot be perturbed have a greater survival value. Therefore, Goodwin's theory cannot be well applied to biological systems.

Enhanced Speed of Chemical Communication: L. E. Scriven and R. Blumenthal

That chemical wave propagation is faster than diffusion was shown by Beck and Váradi (1972), who, by following the movement of

TABLE 1

Conduction Velocities for Several Chemical Waves
[Blumenthal]

Wave	Cm/sec
Slime mold amoeba movement (Gerisch, 1972)	10^4
Belousov-Zhabotinsky reaction (Winfree, 1972)	10^{-2}
Activation spread on iron wire in nitric acid (Bonhoeffer, 1953)	120
Conduction of impulse in squid giant axon (Hodgkin, 1964)	2500

the front of a pH indicator, observed that the rate of movement of a color front in the Belousov-Zhabotinsky reaction was 200 times greater than the rate of diffusion of hydrogen ions. The propagation velocity of a small-amplitude chemical wave of sinusoidal form is given by the product of its wavelength and the frequency of the source exciting the wave (Gmitro and Scriven, 1966). In general, the derived expressions for the wave propagation velocity as a function of reaction rate constants, diffusion constants, and local concentrations of the chemical species participating in the reaction become unwieldy. In a limited range of excitation frequencies and with one chemical species participating in the reaction, however, one can derive a very simple expression for the wave propagation velocity: the square root of the product of the rate constant of the reaction and the diffusion constant of the chemical species. By taking 10^2/sec for the reaction rate constant and 10^{-6} cm^2/sec for the diffusion constant, the wave propagation velocity will be 10^{-2} cm/sec. In the same system without a wave-propagating mechanism but with a concentation difference of 1 mole/cm^3 over 1 cm, the diffusion velocity will be approximately 10^{-6} cm/sec. Thus, the chemical wave enhances the speed of mass transport 10,000-fold. The wave for a one-species system, however, attenuates very rapidly. In the present example, the wave decreases in 1 cm to 5×10^{-5} of its original amplitude. On the other hand, Gmitro and Scriven (1966) have shown that, with more participating species, one can get wave propagation of considerable velocity without attenuation. Table 1 gives experimentally observed conduction velocities for several chemical waves, and shows that, even though chemical propagation is much faster than diffusion, it is still much slower than an action potential.

Multiple Modes of Communication: A. Katchalsky, L. E. Scriven, and R. Blumenthal

Chemical signals can be propagated as concentration waves traveling at speeds greater than those allowed by transport alone, i.e., diffusion (Gmitro and Scriven, 1966; Othmer and Scriven, 1971). Such concentration waves could provide large numbers of parallel signal transmission channels between cells in a network. "Cells" in the physical sense refer to regions of comparatively rapid transport surrounded by envelopes having high resistance to transport. To the extent a system is compartmentalized into cells, transport can be made to depend on the number of cells to be traversed rather than on actual distance. This results from localized routes being established through particular sequences of cells. Analysis of such systems permits cell size, shape, and contact configurations to be replaced by numbers and relationships of cells in terms of collective behavior (see the matrix of elements and matrix relations discussed below). Othmer and Scriven (1974) have studied nonlinear aspects of reaction and transport control of dynamic pattern in networks of cells. At the Work Session, Scriven and Katchalsky emphasized the need to devote much more effort to the development of chemical probes that can be used in biological systems at the cellular level.

The interacting domains of neurons, glia, and intercellular space provide a substrate for the innumerable interactive flows of ionic and organic components. Patterns of increasing complexity then emerge that may lead to what Schmitt describes as "connectionist mechanisms . . . based on 'physical chemical changes induced by graded wave processes passing in specific spatio-temporal patterns across sheets of nerve cells' " (Schmitt and Samson, 1969).

How could a macromolecular structure respond to a specific chemical wave out of the innumerable chemical waves that might be propagated? One possibility is that a given macromolecule may respond resonantly only to a particular wavelength or frequency. Generally, we think of specificity in terms of the relatively fixed three-dimensional structure of molecules, as, for example, in recognition sites of enzymes for substrates and receptors for transmitters. The chemical wave hypothesis suggests the alternative of a dynamic macromolecular process that is responsive to the frequency and phase of a chemical wave. As stimulating as this concept is, the case necessitating its invocation has not yet been established.

Kauffman (1972) proposed a model for contact inhibition of cell movement based on a similar notion, in which extension and retraction of pseudopodia are controlled by some underlying continuous biochemical oscillator. Coupling oscillators in two cells by diffusion of oscillator variables should lead to transient damping or contact paralysis when the two are out of phase. It should yield no contact paralysis when portions of two cells in the same phase are apposed, because the diffusive coupling term, according to Fick's law, becomes zero when both copies of the oscillator are identical for all variables. Kauffman (1974) found precisely these results on circular propagation of blebs on neighboring dissociated newt blastula cells. His model would allow stable or transient contact paralysis, asymmetric paralysis of only one interacting partner, and even contact facilitation of movement as properties of coupled nonlinear oscillators.

III. CONTINUITY-DISCONTINUITY PROBLEMS

Continuous Systems

Biochemical Limit-Cycle Oscillations: R. Blumenthal and V. Rowland

The Belousov-Zhabotinsky reaction demonstrates the emergence from an initially homogeneous solution of both spatial (band and spiral) and temporal (oscillatory) patterns. Oscillations are a temporal dynamic pattern and appear in living systems at widely distinct levels and with widely different properties and frequency values.

In Table 2 are presented data concerning oscillations recorded at the molecular level (oscillations of concentrations of metabolites of enzyme reaction pathways) and at the cellular level (endogenous pacemakers). In this section on continuous systems, the focus is on oscillations of intermediates in the glycolytic pathway observed in cell-free extracts of yeast (Chance et al., 1964) and cardiac muscle as well as in a reconstructed glycolytic system (Hess and Boiteux, 1968). In all the systems investigated, the concentrations of the intermediates of glycolysis were found to oscillate with the same frequency as nicotinamide adenine dinucleotide. This was the first demonstration of periodic operation in an enzymic system.

Sustained oscillations in catalytic systems have been the subject of a number of theoretical studies. By analyzing the matrix of rate equations, Hearon (1953) has shown that periodic reactions cannot

TABLE 2

Periods of Sustained Oscillations in Chemical and Biological Systems [Blumenthal]

System	Min
Beats of embryonic heart cells in culture (DeHaan and Sachs, 1972)	10^{-2}
Parabolic burster of the sea hare *Aplysia californica* (Strumwasser, 1968)	1
Belousov-Zhabotinsky reaction (Zhabotinsky, 1967)	1
Glycolytic oscillations (Chance et al., 1964, 1965; Hess and Boiteux, 1968)	2-5
Dictyostelium discoideum aggregation (Robertson and Cohen, 1972)	5
Cytoplasmic pumping in *Physarum polycephalum* (Kauffman)*	1
The mitotic cycle in *Physarum polycephalum* (Kauffman and Wille, 1974)†	600-660

*S. Kauffman, private communication.
†According to Kauffman the mitotic "clock" in *Physarum* is a continuous biochemical oscillator that gates mitosis and DNA replications; the latter processes are not themselves causal parts of the oscillator.

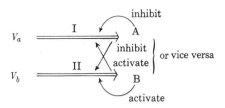

Figure 27. A. A generalized scheme of two coupled (bio)chemical reactions (I and II) that produce oscillations. A and B are chemicals; V_a and V_b = rates of production of A and B.

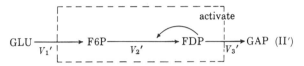

Figure 27. B. Chemical reactions and their rates (V_1', V_2', and V_3') in the glycolytic pathway. GLU = glucose; F6P = fructose-6-phosphate; FDP = fructose-1,6-diphosphate; GAP = glyceraldehyde-3-phosphate. [Higgins, 1964]

occur in a closed system described by *linear* differential equations. Higgins (1964) applied the general principles of oscillator dynamics to chemical systems by stating reaction pathways necessary for a chemical system to exhibit oscillatory behavior (Figure 27A). Let A and B represent chemicals whose net rates of production (V_a, V_b) are determined by arbitrary sets of pathways labeled I and II. The neuroscientist will see in the reciprocal interactions the similarity of Higgins' diagram to excitatory and inhibitory neural control circuits. Oscillations can exist if (1) one of the chemicals activates its own production, (2) one of the chemicals inactivates its own production, and (3) there is cross-coupling of opposite character. In the last case, increased B activates the production of A, and, conversely, increased A inhibits the production of B.

Higgins applied this model to a glycolytic pathway involving the product-activated reaction of the enzyme phosphofructokinase (Figure 27B). Substituting fructose-6-phosphate (F6P) for A and fructose-1,6-diphosphate (FDP) for B, $V_a = V_1 - V_2$ and $V_b = V_2 - V_3$. FDP activation of the kinase increases V_2, thus decreasing V_a and increasing V_b and satisfying the oscillatory coupling conditions. Sustained oscillations occur according to the reaction scheme if the glucose concentration is maintained constant. Figure 27C shows that a continuous energy source permits the system to be open and far from equilibrium.

Under the usual experimental conditions, the glucose concentration decays, and the oscillations disappear. However, Hess and Boiteux (1968), by continuously injecting glycolytic substrates, showed sustained oscillation in cell-free extracts of glycolytic systems.

62

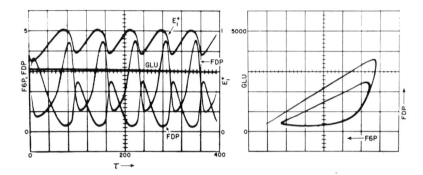

Figure 27. C. Sustained oscillations in glycolysis under condition of virtually constant glucose concentration. The right-hand figure shows the associated phase plane trajectory. The concentration scales are indicated in normalized units; both enzymes have a scale of 1.0. The time scale is in normalized units. E_1^+ represents an activated form of phosphofructokinase. [Higgins, 1964]

Recently, Goldbeter and Lefever (1972) introduced an allosteric mechanism for the phosphofructokinase reaction. The system is described by three distinct and independent parameters that can be interpreted in terms of the molecular properties and interactions of enzyme, substrate, and product. Cyclic AMP, the activator of phosphofructokinase, may play a role in the control of limit-cycle behavior.

Most, if not all, demonstrated biochemical oscillations have periods too long for comparison with the most familiar brain wave frequencies. Intermediate between these two periods (0.02-0.5 sec for the EEG and 1-5 min for chemical oscillations—see Table 2) are the oscillations of local oxygen recordable by the technique of polarography (platinum cathode). The period of oxygen oscillations from various sources ranges from 6 to 12 sec (frequencies from 5-10/min), but this does not correlate with the respiratory rhythm and appears to be a basic oscillation of complex origin. In view of the limit-cycle characteristics of oscillating chemical systems, it is conceivable that a mechanism of this kind may be going on in brain, and the frequency differences are reflecting special properties of an organized cellular system in a multiionic matrix as compared to a simpler diffusion-reaction system like that of Chance and his co-workers (1964) and others.

Rowland has observed, in confirmation of earlier reports, slow oscillatory phenomena that are attributed to "available" oxygen (aO_2) in tissue adjacent to a platinum cathode. Slow CNS oscillations are also reported in microthermal measurements. (These are summarized in Table 3.) Interested in clarifying their possible contribution in steady

TABLE 3

Sampling of Literature on Slow Oscillations in CNS: Some Authors Emphasize
Independence From Cardiovascular and Respiratory Rhythms [Rowland]

Variable	Authors	Frequency (cycles/min)	Period (sec)	Amplitude	Comments
aO_2	Clark and Mishrahy, 1957	8-10	7.5-6	Unstated	Awake cats. Changes with seizures, drugs, etc. Steady potential shifts not oscillatory unless dc offsets high; this confirmed by Rowland.
	Davies and Bronk, 1957	5	12	Estimated 8% of standing O_2 tension near pial artery; 30-50% of tension near pial vein	Cat under moderate to light pentobarbital anesthesia. Oscillations generally independent of blood pressure and respiratory rhythms. Authors rejected metabolic origin in favor of some vascular surging.
	Travis and Clark, 1965	5-10	6-12	0.1 μA change in polarograph current	Awake conditioned cats. Background cycling with acquired conditioned changes.
	Clark and Sachs, 1968	10	6	Unstated	Awake cat. Averaged responses to tone.
	Gijsbers and Melzack, 1967	0.8, 8.5	48, 7	2% change in O_2 cathode current	Awake cat. Background cycling and changes with visual stimulation.
	Rowland (unpublished)	18 / 5.7 / 7	3.3 / 10.5 / 8.5	2-5% of O_2 change from normal O_2 levels to complete asphyxia	Awake rat. / Cat; light pentobarbital. / Awake cat. Steady potential shifts independent of aO_2 (see Clark and Mishrahy, 1957).
Temperature	Melzack and Casey, 1967	3-4 / 6-8	20-15 / 10-7.5	0.001°C	Cat; light pentobarbital.
	Rowland (unpublished)	5-6	12-10	0.002°C	Awake implanted rat. Steady potential shifts independent of thermal oscillations and shifts. (Confirms Kawamura and Sawyer, 1965; Kawamura et al., 1966.)
Electro-corticogram	Aladjalova, 1964	0.5-15	30-4	50-1000 μV	Crickets to mammals. Called infraslow potentials. Many drug effects. Platinum electrodes may have reflected aO_2 rather than shift in steady-state level of voltage generators.
	Norton and Jewett, 1965	0.5-1.5 / 3-5 / 8-14	30-10 / 20-12 / 7.5-4	100-400 μV / 100-500 μV / 100-800 μV	Cat; light anesthesia, pentobarbital and other drugs. Also conscious animals.

64

potential measurements, Rowland observed that the steady potential shift time courses are generally not directly linked to aO_2 and temperature and, thus, he did not pursue the matter further. There is renewed interest in them, however, in light of the many demonstrations of slow chemical oscillations described above. Are thermal and aO_2 oscillations possible counterparts in the brain parenchyma of chemical dynamic patterns in the same sense that the NAD-NADH system* of Chance is?

Table 3 also indicates, in addition to slow oscillations of aO_2 and temperature, slow oscillations of voltage reported in the literature. In this brief review no attempt has been made to survey the more recent literature. All of these scattered observations deserve renewed and intensive investigation in terms of the general dynamics of temporal pattern (oscillation) specified by Katchalsky and others.

Field Concept in Biological Development

Although a developing tissue consists of discrete elements (cells), the introduction of the field concept in developmental biology leads to the description of the process in terms of a continuous system. As noted previously, a "field" has been defined in embryology by Wolpert (1969) as "that region in which all cells have their positional information specified with respect to the same set of points." Continuity is ensured by communication pathways for electrical signals (ions) and metabolites through cell junctions. Cellular coupling is widespread in the embryo during early embryogenesis but decreases during organogenesis (Loewenstein, 1968a; DeHaan and Sachs, 1972). In a formal treatment of developing fields, Robertson and Cohen (1972) introduced a cell state vector that is grouped into two subvectors:

$$S = (S_1, S_2) \tag{14}$$

Whereas the components of S_1 are those needed to specify cell types, the progress of differentiation among them, and the operation of basic processes, the components of S_2 pertain to the operation of the developmental control system per se. Many possibilities for the control variables, S_2, have been considered over the years. According to Turing (1952), the control variables may be construed as a set of substances

---

*NAD-NADH system = nicotinamide adenine dinucleotide-reduced nicotinamide adenine dinucleotide system.

(morphogens), e.g., $S_2 = (C_1, C_2 \ldots C_m)$. Alternatively, various kinds of activity, e.g., rate of differentiation (Huxley and De Beer, 1934), threshold of response (Webster, 1966), and temporal organization of cells (Goodwin and Cohen, 1969) have been taken as a basis for control.

Robertson and Cohen (1972) proposed an equation of motion for the cell state vector to describe the dynamics of coupled cells:

$$\dot{S} = F(S) \tag{15}$$

where F is a function of S. The authors show that Equation 15 can exhibit instability under conditions in which development occurs.

Discontinuous Systems: R. Blumenthal

Membrane Dynamics

Blumenthal and his collaborators (1970) analyzed a molecular mechanism underlying the dynamic behavior of excitable membranes in terms of the unstable transitions exhibited by dynamic patterns (termed "dissipative instabilities" by the authors). They considered the analogy of membrane excitation to the control of regulatory proteins by allosteric ligands (Changeux, 1966, 1969). More precisely, chemical excitation (neurotransmitter-receptor interaction) was viewed as an allosteric interaction (Koshland, 1963; Monod et al., 1963) between two different classes of specific membrane "ligands": the chemical effector (neurotransmitter) and the charged permeant (Na^+, K^+, Cl^-, etc.)(Changeux and Podleski, 1968; Changeux and Thiéry, 1968; Changeux, 1969).

A striking physical property of excitable membranes is their dependence on the nonequilibrium character of the environment in which they function (Katchalsky and Spangler, 1968). Electrical excitation is coupled with a passive translocation of ions through the membrane that propagates the electrical signal. This system irreversibly dissipates the electrochemical energy accumulated in the ionic gradient established across the membrane with repolarization. Thus, membrane excitability can be viewed in the conceptual framework of Prigogine (1969) based on the thermodynamics of open systems whose spatio-temporal organization is coupled with energy dissipation.

The molecular organization of the membrane that exhibits the dynamic properties postulated by Blumenthal and his collaborators (1970) is as follows:

1. An excitable membrane is considered to be an open isothermal lattice system placed between two baths of different electrochemical potentials (environmental asymmetry) that create a passive net flux of the permeating species, p, across the lattice (Changeux, 1969).

2. The membrane lattice is made up of equivalent lipoproteic units, or protomers, specialized in the selective translocation of p. Each protomer carries at least two distinct specific sites for p: one on the inner face of the membrane, the other on its outer face. The permeant both binds and permeates across the membrane, and transport takes place by a "jump" of p from one site to the other. The theory holds when the subunits are considered to be "channels" as well as "carriers."

3. At least two conformations, S and R, are reversibly attainable by each protomer, and both the affinity and the permeability of p are altered when there is a transition from one conformation to another. As a convention, the R state will be more permeable and present a higher affinity for p than the S state.

4. Cooperative interactions are established between protomers within the membrane lattice through a conformational coupling (Changeux et al., 1967; Changeux, 1969), and there is no obligatory requirement for a continuous lattice structure throughout the membrane. The protomers might be organized in dispersed clusters or patches as long as they interact in sufficiently large numbers (see discussion in "Terminology and Essential Features" above).

5. There exists, on both sides of the membrane, a physical medium referred to as an "equilibration layer" (Tasaki, 1968) in which the activity and diffusion of the ligand might be different both from that in the bulk solution and from that in the membrane. In this layer, the concentration of the ligand depends on (1) its rate of adsorption on the membrane surface, (2) its rate of transport across the membrane imposed by the gradient, and (3) its rate of diffusion from the bulk solution. The various states of the protomers (in the absence of interactions with other protomers) are depicted in Figure 28.

The dynamics of membrane permeation were calculated by the method of Hill and Kedem (1967) for transport of nonelectrolytes through a membrane lattice. The kinetics of permeation, superimposed on those of the cooperative conformational change, lead to striking

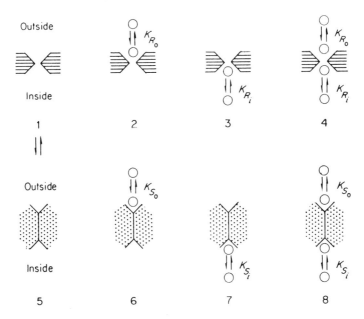

Figure 28. The eight possible states of the membrane protomers. Dots, the transported solute. In the R conformation of the protomer, the solute is both bound and transported. In the S conformation, the solute is bound but not transported. K_{R_o}, K_{R_i}, K_{S_o}, and K_{S_i} are the equilibrium constants for adsorption-desorption of the solute on the outer and inner site of protomers in the R or S state. [Blumenthal et al., 1970]

nonlinear phenomena. Blumenthal and his collaborators (1970) based their calculations, for the sake of simplicity, on a lattice of protomers, using the molecular field (or Bragg-Williams) approximation (Strässler and Kittel, 1965). Blumenthal (1973) has shown that the membrane exhibits the same type of dynamic behavior when the subunits are organized in oligomeric clusters (e.g., tetramers). In Figure 29, the flow through the dynamic membrane is plotted against the concentration gradient of the permeant. A pattern of negative slope permeability appears, a phenomenon familiar in membrane electrical excitability (Cole, 1968). Whereas in electrically excitable systems the negative slope is brought to light by means of a voltage clamp experiment (Hodgkin and Huxley, 1952), in this case a "concentration clamp" experiment is needed to verify the prediction that this model membrane system is excitable.

Interesting properties emerge when the flow through this nonlinear membrane is coupled with a diffusional flow (Figure 30). Assume that there is an unstirred layer apposing the membrane where

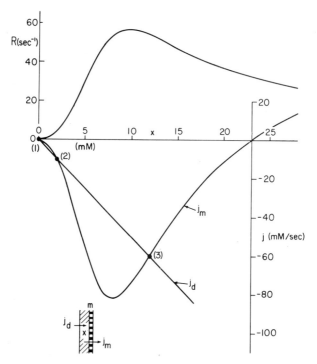

Figure 29. The nonlinear membrane flow (j_m) and the diffusional flow (j_d) into the unstirred layer are plotted concomitantly with the "permeability" (R) as a function of the concentration in the unstirred layer (X, see inset). (1), (2), and (3) represent steady states satisfying Equation 17. [Blumenthal]

the concentration of permeant x is varying (Figure 30A). Two flow processes then participate in the change of x: the nonlinear membrane flow j_m and a simple diffusional flow j_d. Then,

$$\frac{dx}{dt} = j_m - j_d \tag{16}$$

and at a steady state

$$j_m = j_d \tag{17}$$

In Figure 29 j_m and j_d are plotted as a function of x for a given set of concentrations in the bulk solutions. Three steady states are given by the intersections of j_m and j_d, owing to different possible solutions of the nonlinear kinetic equations.

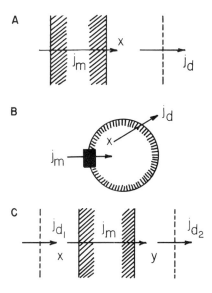

Figure 30. Representation of schemes in which flows are coupled according to Equations 16 and 18. A and C. The diffusional flows (j_d, j_{d_1}, j_{d_2}) are in series with the nonlinear membrane flow (j_m) and changes occur in the concentrations of the transported species (x and y) in the unstirred layers. B. The nonlinear flow (j_m) through a membrane pump site in *parallel* with the flow (j_d) through a leak site produces changes in the overall concentration of the transported species (x) in the cell. [Blumenthal]

Analysis of these steady states shows that the two outer points, 1 and 3, in Figure 29 are stable, while the midpoint, 2, is unstable. Thus, a given threshold signal makes the system jump from one flow or concentration pattern through the unstable point to the other state. In this sense, Prigogine regards excitability as a jump from one dissipative steady state (which is the branch of solutions of kinetic equations that cannot be continuously extrapolated to equilibrium) to another that is closer to equilibrium. The "phase transition" is, therefore, not within the membrane but within the transition from one flow process to the other.

The emergent properties of coupled flow processes can be shown in a single cell with a heterogeneous membrane, i.e., a membrane with different transport and receptor sites (Grundfest, 1966). If the membrane has pump sites parallel to leaks, the concentration within a cell x will be determined by the steady-state coupling of j_m and j_d (Figure 30B). Again, there may be three steady levels for x under a given set of external constraints. If x is an inducer for development that acts only at a certain threshold level, an external transient signal can switch the levels of x.

The Blumenthal-Changeux-Lefever model introduces unstirred layers in which the concentrations of x and y vary as shown in Figure 30C. According to this model,

$$\frac{dx}{dt} = -j_{d_1} + j_m \tag{18}$$

$$\frac{dy}{dt} = -j_m - j_{d_2}$$

If the properties of the unstirred layers are asymmetric, one can show in this simple system the emergence of concentration oscillations (Blumenthal, 1973).

In another example, one can demonstrate two cells that are initially uncoupled. Only the processes j_{d_1} and j_{d_2} are operative, and they will go to equilibrium with the external environment. If an external signal introduces junctional coupling, producing a flow of the type j_m, an oscillating pattern will emerge. This model may be applied to Loewenstein's (1968a) system, in which calcium is both actively transported out of cells and involved in inducing junctional coupling. If one applies this concept to an array of cells, an electrical signal may cause calcium activation, which in turn may cause an overall oscillatory response in terms of the calcium concentration changes in the cells.

Endogenous Pacemaker Cells

The addition of sugars to a suspension of yeast cells, *Saccharomyces carlsbergensis,* causes, after transition to anaerobiosis, characteristic oscillations in the redox state of nicotinamide adenine nucleotides and in the concentrations of glycolytic intermediates (Betz and Chance, 1965). As discussed previously (see pages 60 to 64), the primary pacemaker is believed to be the phosphofructokinase reaction. The oscillations are then transferred to other reactions by means of the fluctuating levels of metabolites and adenine nucleotides. Recently, Becker and Betz (1972) observed that the frequency of oscillations of anaerobic nicotinamide adenine dinucleotides following the addition of fructose is 1.5 to 7.0 times slower than that following the addition of glucose. They pinpointed membrane transport as the controlling pacemaker of glycolysis in *S. carlsbergensis.*

The best-studied endogenous pacemaker in the nervous system is the "parabolic burster," a cell of the parietovisceral ganglion of the sea hare, *Aplysia californica* (Strumwasser, 1965). This cell, as discussed by Lickey (1969), exhibits spontaneous patterned activity on a time scale of minutes, with cycles of bursting and hyperpolarization as well as circadian oscillations in the spike frequency.

After blocking the parabolic burster spike discharges with tetrodotoxin, Strumwasser (1967, 1968) found that spontaneous oscillations of the membrane potential still occur between −30 mV and −65 mV, with a rhythm similar to the burst rhythm. Strumwasser believes that an electrogenic sodium pump is involved in the mechanism of the cell's sustained periodic activity. These are only two of the multitude of autonomously periodic processes known in the biological field (see also Bruce, 1960; Aschoff, 1965; Pittendrigh, 1974).

"Cooperative" Pacemaker Assemblies

What phenomena may arise from the interaction of whole populations of periodic processes? What is the best way to recognize and analyze a multioscillator community and to investigate its integrative mechanisms? Many examples of synchronization of populations of spontaneous pacemakers have been observed, e.g., the tissue-culture experiments of chick embryo cells (DeHaan, 1967), the hagfish heart (Jensen, 1966), the pulsations of coelenterates including jellyfish (Bullock and Horridge, 1965), and the synchronization of flashing in Southeast Asian fireflies (Buck and Buck, 1966).

Van der Pol and Van der Mark (1928) constructed a model for a beating heart from three separate relaxation oscillators, satisfying the Van der Pol equation. These oscillators correspond to the cardiac sinus, the auricle, and the ventricle. Couplings are then introduced from the sinus to the auricle and to the ventricle that correspond to the real heart. The entire system is represented by a set of six dynamic equations, and the solutions correspond, in effect, to an electrocardiogram. By modifying the parameters and couplings appropriately, the model electrocardiogram can be matched to real electrocardiograms of normal and pathological conditions of the heart.

Wiener (1958) explored the notion that the human alpha rhythm might reflect the cooperative behavior of myriads of individual oscillatory processes, i.e., the population of spontaneously active neurons statistically firing in concert. Because autonomous pacemaker cells have not been discovered in the vertebrate central nervous system, this picture of the brain is not very convincing (cf. the Elul model on page 97). Wiener's mathematical approach to mutual synchronization, however, pertains to other biological rhythms, for example, the pulsating jellyfish, which has multiple potential pacemakers in the marginal ganglia or nerve rings (Bullock and Horridge, 1965). These nerve rings reside within the conducting system, accessible to impulses that fire them and reset their rhythm. According to Bullock and Horridge (1965): "Pacemaking is handed around from one to the other, assuring the fastest rhythm available. The pacemakers are also, irreciprocally, accessible to influence from other conducting systems and from sense organs; they are internal clocks subject to modification by adequate phasic and tonic stimuli."

Mutual synchronization of populations of pacemakers obeying nonlinear dissipative dynamics appears appropriate for applying Katchalsky's concept of "cooperative nonequilibrium phenomena." Sastre (1972) defines cooperativity for such systems by making an analogy with the notion used in the Blumenthal-Changeux-Lefever model of cooperativity among protomers in a macromolecule or a membrane (see pages 65 to 70). The change in free energy corresponding to the transition (and hence the probability of the transition's occurring) from the S to the R conformation is dependent on the number of units already in state R. By analogy, it is assumed that the probability of a given endogenously active neuron's exhibiting a given pattern of activity is modified by the number of neurons already exhibiting that particular behavior (see Bennett below). In other words, the more units whose pacemaker potentials are entrained via electrotonic junctions to the pacemaker, the faster is the recruitment of other units oscillating at different frequencies. When groups of pacemaker neurons are isolated, they might fire at different frequencies, but, when interconnected, they are entrained by the fastest unit among them, provided that their native (free-running) rhythms are sufficiently close or the entraining stimulus sufficiently large.* This produces a global coordinated oscillation. Spike electrogenesis is important to reset the rhythm and to synchronize neurons coupled by junctions with too high an attenuation ratio to permit entrainment to their pacemaker potentials. In terms of the cooperative membrane paradigm for the S to

*The pacemaker hypothesis, i.e., that a whole assembly of oscillators are driven by those cells having the most rapid spontaneous frequency, has been advanced so often as to become dogma (DeHaan, 1967). Recently, however, DeHaan and Sachs (1972) have fused isolated beating heart muscle cells in culture in order to determine whether the cell with the faster rate would set the rate of the pair. Of the 37 cell pairs studied only 14 turned out to obey the pacemaker hypothesis.

R transition, the R state would relate to those units that are in phase (entrained), whereas the S state would relate to those that lag behind. Sastre (1972) attempted to apply these notions to patterned behavior in small neuronal systems of invertebrates, as in the cardiac ganglion of the shrimp squilla (Watanabe et al., 1967).

Organizing Waves in Neural Networks

Neural networks have been a biomathematician's delight since the days of McCulloch and Pitts (1943), and real nerve nets can be found in coelenterates (Bullock and Horridge, 1965). Originally thought to be a syncytium, the coelenterate nerve net was shown by Pantin (1952) to be composed of contiguous rather than continuous neurons, at least in the mesenteric net of the sea anemone *Metridium*. Interactions between neurons occur where they meet in crossing, i.e., at synapses. Although the nerve nets are apparently randomly organized, they are capable of some integrative activity and of discrimination of temporal pattern in input sequences (Fehmi and Bullock, 1967).

Josephson and his co-workers (1961), simulating a diffusely conducting system based on coelenterate nerve nets, elucidated electrotonic spread in living nerve nets. A large ratio of transmissive to nontransmissive junctions or a large number of junctions per conducting element lead both to a greater relative distance of spread and to a greater variability in the localization and strength of spread. (For comparison, see Othmer and Scriven's finding, discussed above, on the way the number and relationships of cells determine their collective behavior in chemodiffusional compartmental networks.)

Beurle (1956) characterized nerve cells capable of regenerating impulses by a single scalar state variable of "activity." This included a measurable electrical output, excitatory and inhibitory interactions, threshold phenomena, time lags, and spatial distributions of connections. He studied the behavior of such cells in masses sufficiently large to, permit replacing individual cell properties and interactions by distribution functions, leading to nonlinear partial differential integral equations. These equations actually describe interfering transformation and transport in a system essentially made up of one type of compound. Moreover, they are generically related to the systems in Turing's approach to morphogenesis.

The mass of cells is then capable of supporting various forms of activity including plane waves, spherical and circular waves, and vortex effects (see the discussion above on the Belousov-Zhabotinsky reaction). The wave may be initiated in the cell mass by a number of individual stimuli for which the cells demonstrate a certain threshold. Because the threshold depends on cell properties, the cell mass may be made to act as an on-off switch by altering the threshold (see the discussion above on "local control" by Othmer and Scriven). Beurle (1956) compares the switching of waves with the shifting of attention in living organisms. If some property of individual cells (e.g., size, extent of axon or dendrite structure, or threshold) changes with repeated use, the cell mass may modify its response according to past experience. Even by taking a very simple arrangement of the cell mass, Beurle can demonstrate such emergent properties as trial and error learning, conditioned responses, and the ability of the organ or organism to regenerate internally a sequence of past events.

Models of Excitatory and Inhibitory Interactions in Neural Tissue

The "neuron doctrine," which classically describes discrete synaptic contacts among clearly separated elements, is basic to the connectionist view. The dynamic pattern concept does not contradict this view and, in fact, is compatible if rates of change in neuronal activity are regarded as the "flows" dynamically maintaining a pattern. An example of what might be called a connectionist model comparable to a dissipative structure has been worked out mathematically by Wilson and Cowan (1972). By postulating the operation of a neural net based on separate populations of excitatory (E) and inhibitory (I) neurons, with random spatial interconnection, they developed a two-variable treatment of neural activity (i.e., $E(t)$ = the proportion of excitatory cells firing per unit time and $I(t)$ = the proportion of inhibitory cells firing per unit time) and arrived at the following equations for the rate of change of these variables:

$$\tau_e \frac{dE}{dt} = -E + (k_e - r_e E)S_e(c_1 E - c_2 I + P) \tag{19}$$

$$\tau_i \frac{dI}{dt} = -I + (k_i - r_i I)S_i(c_3 E - c_4 I + Q)$$

where τ signifies the time delays of the respective populations; r, their refractory periods; S, subpopulation response functions; k, maximum values of the response functions; c, connectivity coefficients; and P and Q, the external input to excitatory and inhibitory subpopulations, respectively.

They analyzed these equations qualitatively, using the E, I phase plane. Equations for the isoclines corresponding to $dE/dt = 0$ and $dI/dt = 0$ are

$$c_2 I = c_1 E - S_e^{-1}\left(\frac{E}{k_e - r_e E}\right) + P \text{ for } \frac{dE}{dt} = 0 \qquad (20)$$

$$c_3 E = c_4 I + S_i^{-1}\left(\frac{I}{k_i - r_i I}\right) - Q \text{ for } \frac{dI}{dt} = 0$$

A typical plot (Figure 31B) shows three steady-state solutions corresponding to the three intersections of the two curves: the outer intersects, (+) and (+), are stable, whereas the intermediate intersect, (−), is unstable. As is directly evident from the graph, the two stable steady states correspond, respectively, to (1) high proportions of both excitatory and inhibitory neurons and (2) a low proportion of both.

The system as defined at the intermediate state responds to small perturbations by moving to one or the other stable state point. Alternatively, a threshold input to the system in one stable state drives the system into its other state, with a "jump" through the transition region. This model is analogous to a dynamic pattern (dissipative structure) defined by Katchalsky (see above). The transition across the range of instability creates two different temporal and spatial organizations of the neural network. In this sense, there are two different

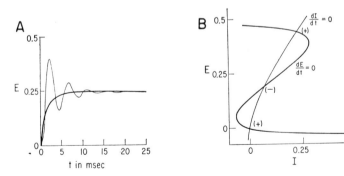

Figure 31. A. The proportion of excitatory (E) neurons firing per unit time as a function of time obtained by solving Equation 19. B. A phase plane diagram of proportions of excitatory (E) and inhibitory (I) neurons firing per unit time, according to Equation 20. (+) denotes stability and (−) instability of the steady state. [Wilson and Cowan, 1972]

"flow" patterns, each requiring energy. This energy has to be continuously supplied since it is also being continuously lost from the system, hence, the use of the term "dissipative." The energy source is not identified by Wilson and Cowan, but it presumably relates to the metabolic exchanges characterizing all neural function at background or resting level as well as at varying levels of activity.

Wilson and Cowan have extended their model to multiple ranges of steady states that agree with Katchalsky's concept of a spectral hierarchy of dynamic patterns. Also, as a function of external inputs, the model of Wilson and Cowan exhibits hysteresis that is of interest in the theory of short-term memory. The transient behavior of this neural model, exhibiting damped oscillatory response to brief external inputs, compares favorably with averaged evoked potentials observed neurophysiologically.

A second form of temporal behavior, perhaps of greater functional significance than the damped oscillation, is the limit cycle. Under certain conditions, as when the interactions within the excitatory subpopulation greatly exceed those within the inhibitory subpopulation, only one intersection of the isoclines occurs, reflecting a single steady state for the system located in the transition region. Perturbations displacing the system from this steady state will cause it to develop a stable cycling (limit cycle) around its former single steady state. The limit cycle may also be attained when the system approaches its steady state from any other initial condition (Glansdorff and Prigogine, 1971).

An important property of the limit cycle is the variation of its frequency directly and monotonically with a specific range of external input. Below this range, limit-cycle activity cannot occur; above it, limit-cycle activity is extinguished. Using the physiological observations of Poggio and Viernstein (1964), Wilson and Cowan propose that their model is compatible with the idea of stimulus intensity being coded into both average spike frequency and periodic modulations of that average. Monotonic increase in frequency over a limited range with input amplitude was also predicted from a similar model by Freeman (1967). It was experimentally demonstrated in the prepiriform cortex by measurement of the change in frequency of average evoked potentials and poststimulus histograms over a range of amplitude of background cortical activity (Freeman, 1968d).

Wilson and Cowan make no special claim regarding the applicability of their model to the electroencephalogram (EEG) but suggest the possibility that the limit-cycle theory may provide a more concrete understanding of it. That external stimulation above threshold is necessary to elicit limit-cycle performance of the system is quite opposite to the conditions favoring elicitation of sustained EEG periodicity. This exception does not hold, however, with periodic stimulation, as in photic driving, which may be very relevant to the model of Wilson and Cowan.

According to Bullock, model systems that take into account fewer element properties than those used by Wilson and Cowan (for example, no inhibition) lead to computer-determined outputs of vast complexity (see the previous section). One does not need many element properties to obtain highly versatile systems. In Bullock's view, increasing knowledge of biological reality may go in two directions in advancing this mode of thinking: it may provide constraints that lead to a reduction in the number of possible operations of a model set, or it may increase even more the possible states of an already unwieldy system.

IV. MIXED SYSTEMS

The Continuity-Discreteness Problem:
V. Rowland

The implications of the dynamic pattern concept discussed in the preceding sections make the division into continuous and discontinuous domains seem arbitrary, helpful as it is for purposes of exposition. The judgment of discreteness and continuity is obviously relative and dependent on the level of spatial or temporal magnitudes under consideration. For example, extracellular space, if conceptualized in a macroscopic context, is a continuous domain. In a microscopic context, however, it is composed of discrete entities whose interrelations give rise to the properties recognized in the macroscopic sense.

Frequently, the nervous system is viewed as a combination of discrete structures (e.g., cells, organelles, and membranes) and a continuous medium (extracellular space). Since the theory of dynamic pattern developed above is shown to apply equally well to discrete element systems and continuous domains, there is no a priori expectation that unique, basic theoretical considerations appear as a result of considering them together, i.e., as mixed systems. However, if it is ultimately shown that the dynamic pattern concept proves parsimonious and generalizable in neuroscience, one possible outcome of considering discrete systems embedded in a continuous system would be the subordination of obvious structural discreteness to a functional one: the spatially discrete elements could be brought to functional continuity (see Wilson and Cowan above) or the structurally continuous medium to functional (dynamic) discontinuity, as exemplified by convection cells or the Belousov-Zhabotinsky effect. If the applicability of this theory to neuroscience is confirmed, it would be expected to change our thinking about the structural criterion for distinguishing continuity from discreteness rather than be abandoned because of this criterion. This problem arose both implicitly and explicitly at the Work Session, the classical structural position being defended as sufficient and the dissipative structure or dynamic pattern position being attacked as unnecessary for understanding the complexity of nervous systems.

How, then, is one to think of continuity and discreteness? What is spatially discrete in system *structure* may be temporally continuous in system *function* and vice versa. Perhaps all the Work Session participants would agree that, no matter how compelling spatial discreteness or continuity may appear in biology, the spatial criterion alone is insufficient for an understanding of a system's operation. What, then, is added with temporal considerations that could not be deduced from spatial organization? We return to the familiar character of dynamics, i.e., material patterns changing in time and the flows of molecules, ions, electric currents, heat, etc., changing in relation to the forces operating amid static structures.

The issue of continuity and discreteness is relative even in the time domain. Although time is generally regarded as continuous, events (which are the only basis for measuring time) need not be. Events can be temporal discontinuities in the same sense that points are spatial discontinuities. The pulse codes produced by trains of action potentials represent discrete patterns in time as well as space. Thus, neither time nor space alone can be the basis of a complete criterion, and, if we adhere preferentially to either of them, we may be confined to clumsy or incomplete descriptions of system operation. It may be argued that this is nothing new; this occurs any time some spatial or other variable is graphed as a function of time. Familiar as it is, the problem has to be reworked in complex systems. Obvious boundaries for discrete elements (exemplified in neuroscience by the neuron doctrine) may be necessary for understanding many properties of the system. However, such element boundaries are not by their "necessity" automatically established as sufficient for understanding all properties of the system.

Functional Boundaries

The ultimate criterion is the character of transitions (boundaries) in a spatiotemporal functioning or operating system. The dynamic pattern concept suggests this in the jump transition through an unstable region, as shown in phase space between two domains which differ qualitatively (i.e., the organizational or hierarchical rules differ for the two domains). The unstable region constitutes a functional equivalent of a boundary between functionally discrete states of a system. This boundary can be quite different from the boundaries recognized either in time or space alone.

"Functional" boundaries will be identifiable in proportion to the sharpness of transition between identifiable states. Such sharpness (rate of change with respect to space and time) is a more operational descriptor than stability-instability because a rapid transition in a complex subsystem may either promote or disrupt stability in the larger system of which it is a component. Thresholds, accelerated chemical interactions based on cooperativity, etc., cannot be judged as stabilizing or destabilizing independently of the overall consequences of their occurrence.

Rapid transitions may be synergistic, as in enzymatic catalysis and action potential propagation, or may be disruptive in large complex systems, as in impulsive behavior in humans or in epilepsy. The latter raises the question whether dynamic patterns can appear so compelling a consequence of complexity in biological systems that they can give rise to maladaptive functioning ("pathologic" dynamic patterns). Because of this possibility, studies in relation to epilepsy and spreading depression were included in the Work Session (see Ferguson and Van Harreveld below).

In the above discussion of a combination of discrete and continuous systems, it is implied that the continuous extracellular medium of brain is homogeneous. The nonhomogeneous structuring of this space, however, and the concept of the "greater membrane" were dealt with at a previous Work Session (Schmitt and Samson, 1969).

Extracellular Microenvironment:
W. R. Adey

Electrical Impedance and Calcium

Adey and his colleagues have taken the electrical impedance of brain tissue as an indication of the state of this extracellular microenvironment, including its responses to altered calcium levels. They have measured impedance in the cerebral cortex in acute experiments (Adey et al., 1969; Adey, 1971b) and in periventricular structures in chronically prepared animals (Wang and Adey, 1969). In both sets of experiments, the increase in calcium concentration in the bathing fluid was approximately 10 times above typical levels of 2.0 mM in cerebrospinal fluid (CSF). Increased ventricular calcium lowered the impedance of periventricular structures in chronic preparations. In acute experiments, however, cortical impedance was raised by added calcium. This divergent action of calcium in acute and chronic experiments may relate to gradual development of an organized tissue-electrode interface in the chronic preparations over a period of about 3 weeks. A similarly inverted pattern developed in the impedance responses of human limbic tissue to decreased CO_2 levels in the first month of electrode implantation and accompanied a gradual rise in base line impedance over that period (Porter et al., 1964).

The greater membrane model (Schmitt and Samson, 1969) proposes polyanionic extensions (which form a suitable substrate for binding calcium and other cations) that may extend into the extracellular space from glial and neuronal surfaces. Although Adey's own studies demonstrate that presumed neuroglial cells are sensitive to extracellular calcium, he emphasized a critical role for calcium on the neuronal membrane. He proposed a model of excitatory regulation in cerebral tissue that would complement synaptic connectivity, hitherto regarded as the exclusive mechanism for information processing in the nervous system. According to this model, a traveling wave of altered Ca^{2+} binding on a macromolecular substrate is "compatible with known rates of decremental conduction in dendrites" (Adey, 1974).

Having shown the effects of calcium on extracellular conductance and on cellular polarization properties, Adey (1971a,b), nevertheless, stressed the need for caution in interpreting the effects of transient topical applications of calcium, with its slow diffusion into cortex. Moreover, effects seen with topical calcium concentrations 20 to 30 times the physiological level may not be useful in modeling physiological functions. In subsequent studies, Kaczmarek and Adey (1973) examined the efflux of $^{45}Ca^{2+}$ and $[^3H]\gamma$-aminobutyric acid (^{3}H-GABA) from superfused cat cortex in response to much smaller increments in unlabeled Ca^{2+} concentration. Increases in Ca^{2+} concentration of the medium resulted in a greater efflux of both $^{45}Ca^{2+}$ and ^{3}H-GABA. The effect of a 1 mM increment in Ca^{2+} concentration was only slightly less than that of a 20 mM increment (Figure 32). Thus, calcium triggers its own release, a phenomenon strongly suggesting cooperative binding and release. Mg^{2+} did not show comparable effects.

Two mechanisms are consistent with the observed kinetics. Classically, the efflux of Ca^{2+} may be limited by the concentration of a free carrier in the membrane. Thus, an increase in the binding of Ca^{2+}, due to increased external Ca^{2+} concentration, results in a net movement of Ca^{2+} carrier to the inside of the membrane where it may rebind to $^{45}Ca^{2+}$ and thence increase $^{45}Ca^{2+}$ efflux. Alternatively, the increase in unlabeled Ca^{2+} may displace $^{45}Ca^{2+}$ bound to polyanionic sites at the surface of the membrane (Hafemann et al., 1969). To be consistent

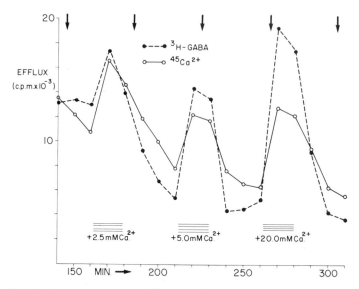

Figure 32. The simultaneous efflux of $^{45}Ca^{2+}$ and ^{3}H-GABA from cat cortex in an experiment in which aminooxyacetic acid (5 mg/kg body wt) had been administered before incubation with ^{3}H-GABA. The superfusion medium contained 2.16 mM Ca^{2+} before increasing the Ca^{2+} concentration by the amounts indicated. Time after the start of superfusion is shown on the abscissa and the arrows indicate administration of gallamine triethiodide to sustain immobilization. [Kaczmarek and Adey, 1973]

with the observed $^{45}Ca^{2+}$ efflux and net Ca^{2+} binding, this second mechanism may take the form

$$Ca^{2+} + {}^{45}Ca\text{-}M^{n-} \rightarrow {}^{45}Ca\text{-}M^{(n-2)-}$$

$$^{45}Ca\text{-}Ca\text{-}M^{(n-2)-} \rightarrow {}^{45}Ca^{2+} + Ca\text{-}M^{n-}$$

where M represents a membrane anionic species and n represents multiple fixed charges. In this way, the efflux of Ca^{2+} from the membrane is proportional to a high power of the bound Ca^{2+} concentration.

Adey also discussed the possibility that the neuron might "determine its own weather" if it possesses the capacity to modify its local environment through opposing actions of divalent cations and dicarboxylic amino acids. This capacity might significantly modify its postsynaptic responsiveness.

In contrast to the data of Eidelberg (1962, 1963), who found no effect of topical calcium on a cortical steady potential that was

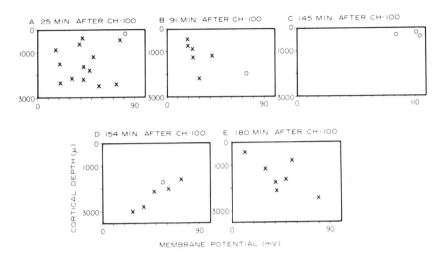

Figure 33. Effect of topical polyanion gel, Chelex-100, on cat cortical membrane potentials plotted against cortical depth. In Track A, neuronal membrane potentials were at first as high as in control cortex but decreased to essentially complete depolarization (Track C). Repolarization first occurred at depths greater than 1500 μM. Mean neuronal membrane potentials: Track A, 42.9 ± 18.1 mV; Track B, 26.2 ± 8.8 mV; Track D, 54.5 ± 9.2 mV; Track E, 43.2 ± 22.9 mV. The t-tests showed no significant differences between these means, nor between them and normal cortex. X = neurons; o = silent cells. [Adey]

highly reactive to potassium, Adey (1971b) reported a decrease of the 10 mV transcortical dc gradient 25 min after application of Ca^{2+} at a 30-fold CSF concentration. This treatment depolarized neurons and "silent" cells and produced EEG seizures. Lower concentrations of topical calcium (at a 20-fold CSF level) were found to hyperpolarize neurons but continued to depolarize "silent" cells. Using vertical microelectrode tracks through the cortex after placing a 10-fold increase of topical Ca^{2+} over several hours, Adey observed increased numbers of hyperpolarized neurons; by contrast, a similar administration of L-glutamic acid produced more depolarized cells.

In the presence of a chelating resin (Chelex-100) that reduces cation concentrations at the brain surface, Adey observed membrane depolarization within 2 hours of application. However, this did not occur with resins presaturated with Ca^{2+} (Figure 33). Therefore, Adey concluded that Ca^{2+} was chelated by the resin and that zero Ca^{2+} concentration depolarized, whereas 10-fold CSF Ca^{2+} concentration hyperpolarized neuronal membranes. He also found that a high Ca^{2+} concentration blocked the capacity of topical L-glutamic acid to depolarize neurons, if the increment in Ca^{2+} concentration preceded glutamic acid addition, but it had little effect after glutamic acid addition.

Somjen and others (Kemény et al., 1961; Hilmy and Somjen, 1968) found that the Mg^{2+} content of CSF and brain extracellular fluid was independent of blood levels and felt that the same was probably true for Ca^{2+}. They interpreted this to mean that an effective blood-brain barrier existed for these divalent cations. Adey concurred, citing the long recovery time (180 or more minutes) required for neuronal membrane potentials from depolarization induced by removal of Ca^{2+} from their environment. His observations with topical chelating resins indicated that recovery took far longer than would be the case for simple diffusion of Ca^{2+} from capillaries over typical intercapillary distances of about 50 μm (Adey, 1971a; Costin et al., 1974). Reappearance of membrane potentials in all cortical layers was associated with intermittent EEG seizures. This slow recovery is in agreement with the rates observed for equilibration with CSF in the dog (Oppelt et al., 1963), but is slower than the rates found in Mg^{2+} deficiency (Woodward and Reed, 1969).

Adey interpreted these effects in terms of the neuron's capacity to modify its local environment through opposing actions of divalent cations and dicarboxylic amino acids. Furthermore, he envisages cooperative processes between divalent cations and membrane surface polyanions and postulates that the latter may be capable of transduction and amplification of electrical signals. Kaczmarek and Adey (1974a,b) have stimulated cat cortex with agar-bridge electrodes, using 1.0 msec pulse trains at 200/sec that produced measured gradients of 20 to 50 mV/cm in the cortex. Although these weak fields are only 10^{-4} to 10^{-5} of the synaptic electric gradient, they elicited a significant efflux of $^{45}Ca^{2+}$ and ^{3}H-GABA from cat cortex (Figure 34). Since these fields are no bigger than the EEG seizure gradient measured in the same tissue, and only 2 to 5 times larger than normal EEG gradients, Adey proposed that this mechanism would enable neurons to sense weak electric fields, and that cortical neuronal assemblies might operate as a system capable of being affected by electrical field gradients.

The role of fluxes of calcium in the extracellular space was questioned. Calcium may pass directly from capillaries (Oppelt et al., 1963) into brain parenchyma or into the CSF via the choroid plexus. Once in the extracellular space, it may be taken up by both neurons and glia. There is histological evidence of its differential concentration

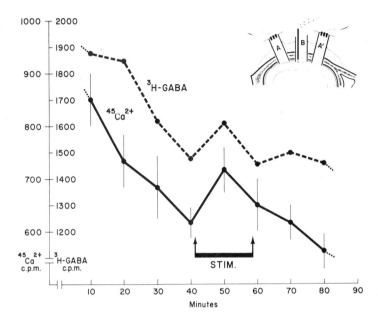

Figure 34. Efflux of $^{45}Ca^{2+}$ and ^{3}H-GABA from superfused cat cortex, and the effect of weak electrical stimulation (200/sec, 1.0 msec pulses) during the period indicated. These plots are of the means with SEM for six experiments. At the top is a diagram of the superfusion cylinder (B) and the agar electrodes (A, A') inserted through trephine holes in the skull and sealed with agar. [Kaczmarek and Adey, 1974b]

in neuroglial cytoplasm (Tarby and Adey, 1967), and calcium's "arriving" in the extracellular space from neuroglia might considerably modify Adey's view of the neuron "determining its own weather." In this case, "the weather" in the intracellular space might be determined by a neuronal-neuroglial interaction rather than by an exclusive neuronal mechanism, but the interaction would still occur across the macromolecular field of the intercellular space. That such an interaction appears likely in the case of potassium was reported by Kuffler and his colleagues (1966) who have noted that neuroglial membranes are sensitive to external potassium concentration changes likely to occur in physiological neuronal responses to excitation.

Katchalsky commented that further studies leading to the identification of the "key" or central controlling changes effected by ions in such complex systems are necessary. For this, he cited the need to develop an improved electrode technology for better time and space resolution of ionic shifts.

Interneuronal Connectivity

Dendrodendritic Junctions: H. Van der Loos

At the light microscope level, Van der Loos (1960) showed that the spatial distribution of dendrodendritic junctions in Golgi preparations of the cerebral neocortex revealed a periodicity that occurred preferentially at about 60, 120, and 180 μ from the cell body (Figure 35). Eighty percent of the contacts were between dendritic segments of the same branching order, and 15% were between dendrites with one order difference. Nothing can be stated about the determinants of this spatial periodicity and about the tendency of segments of the same order to seek out one another. They could be the consequence of structural conditions such as dendrite packing and/or time of contact during dendritic growth. An alternative possibility to this spatial periodicity is the "prepatterning" concept described above (see "Turing's Theory of Morphogenesis"). According to the principles of dynamic pattern formation outlined in Chapter II, the spatial periodicity along the surface of the dendrite might appear at critical nodal points where "junctional material" is accumulated. This spatial periodicity pattern then acts as a functional scaffold for laying a more permanent pattern of dendrodendritic junctions.

The existence, in mammalian neocortex, of dendrodendritic junctions was confirmed by electron microscopy. The junctions have been shown to have three different forms. In one type, Van der Loos (1964, 1968) found interdigitations that considerably enlarge the junctional area between the dendrites (0.5-10 μ^2, mean at 3.0-3.5 μ^2). The cleft between the rigidly parallel membranes often contains, in patches, "interlemmal elements," about 70-A thin structures bridging the interspace. These elements resemble a differentiation that Van der Loos (1963) described in cortical synapses. Sloper (1971) has described, as a second type, synapses between the dendrites and, as a third type, gap junctions (Sloper, 1972). So far, it has been impossible to identify a given junction between dendrites as seen in Golgi preparations with one of the types described in electron microscopy. In view of their frequency of occurrence, it is likely that most of the junctions are of the kind described by Van der Loos. All three types of dendrodendritic connections have been found in other CNS regions in a variety of animals. A form of dendrodendritic apposition, the desmosome, was not found in the cerebral neocortex and was first

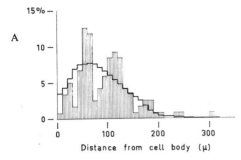

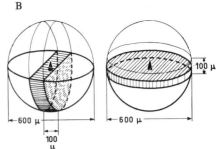

A

C

Distance from cell body (μ)

Distance from cell body (μ)

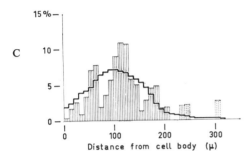

Figure 35. Distribution of dendrite length and of dendrodendritic junctions (DD) as a function of the distance from the perikaryon. Data obtained from 14 pyramids from adult rabbit's first temporal area. A. Data as measured and counted: each 10-μ class contains percentage of the total (basal) dendrite length and of the total number of DD *in that class*. Thus, a "dendrite profile" (heavy line) and DD distribution were determined. Mean basal dendrite length per neuron = ~1500 μ; mean number of DD per neuron = ~8.5. The two distributions are different (pooled data for the 14 neurons; application of χ^2 test: P < 0.02). B. Lower half of the sphere: branching area of basal dendrites. Hatched sections of sphere: parts of the branching area that can be studied in sections suitable for investigation under oil immersion (total magnification, ×2500). *Left:* studied in sections perpendicular to pia; *right:* studied in sections parallel to pia. Black triangle in center of sphere represents perikaryon of pyramidal cell. C. The same distributions as presented in A, but *after correction* for cutting of dendrites by microtome knife needed to obtain the 100-μ thick section in which analysis was carried out. Corrected mean dendrite length per neuron = ~2700 μ; corrected mean number of DD per neuron = ~16.5. When considering that 1 out of 50 neurons captured the Golgi stain and assuming spatial characteristics of stained and unstained neurons identical, one finds the total number of DD on basal dendrites of cortical pyramid = approximately 800. [Van der Loos, 1960]

described by Gray (1961) in the cerebellum. It was also found in other areas and in many species.

It is tempting to assume that the nonsynaptic types of dendrodendritic junctions may be serving as a path for electrotonic spread as described below by Bennett. Bennett and Auerbach (1969) calculated that coupling between nerve cells may occur even in the absence of morphological specialization, such as the reduced cleft width at the junction. Gerard (1942), in his discussion of ephaptic neuronal interaction in general, suggested that, although the action of normal synaptic pathways connot be precluded, such interaction may play a role in the "spread of certain types of waves through neural masses and in synchronization of rhythmic neuron activity."

87

88

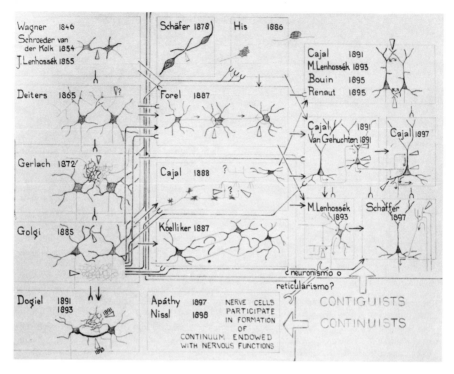

Figure 36. Development of the concept of neuronal connectivity took place in the latter half of the 19th century. Analysis is made from a morphologic point of view. Development begins with R. Wagner's *image of truth* (dendrodendritic junctions at which cell continuity exists). Development ends with Ramón y Cajal's (1897) *images* (axodendritic and axosomatic articulations at which cell contiguity exists; revised law of dynamic polarization). "Ideogenesis" of neuronal connectivity is divided into three stages, each characterized by the emergence of a new concept (chronology is simplified; in the figure, sequencing of concepts prevails over chronology).
I. Period through 1885. *Nerve cell plexuses:* nerve cell interaction through cell continuity. Only concepts stating that nerve cells are central units in performance of nervous system (Purkinje's 1838 postulate) are incorporated.
II. Second half of 1880's. *The independent nerve cell:* neuronal interaction through cell contiguity.
III. 1890's. The synapse and unidirectional signal flow through neuron: "articulations" (Ramón y Cajal) and "useful contacts" (Van Gehuchten) between neurons: "law of dynamic polarization" (Ramón y Cajal and Van Gehuchten). Ideogenesis of nerve cell (see Van der Loos, 1967) took 150 years (1718-1865), whereas that of neuronal connectivity, summarized here, took only 50 years. [Van der Loos]

Van der Loos also demonstrated the interesting historical fact that dendrodendritic connections were postulated, and then discovered, even before the axodendritic and axosomatic synapses that have dominated neural network thinking ever since the 1890's (see Figure 36).

The Autapse

Among the classes of connections Van der Loos described is the contact between the axon and one or more of the dendrites of the same cell, which he calls an autapse (see Figure 37; Van der Loos and Glaser, 1972). Questions were raised concerning the mechanism by which growing neurons avoid, or manage to find, their own processes and the

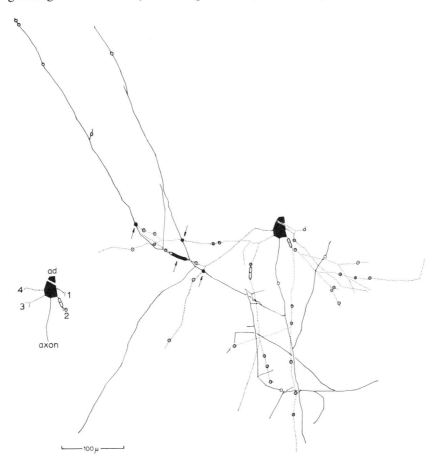

Figure 37. Computer trace of a Golgi-impregnated, autapse-bearing pyramidal cell of rabbit neocortex cerebra. From the cell body emanate the following: *axon,* solid lines; *basal dendrites* 1-4, broken lines; and *apical dendrite* (ad), not traced. Synapses on dendrites made by axons of other Golgi-impregnated cells are shown by ⊙; synapses made by the traced axon upon dendrites of other impregnated cells are shown by ○. Arrows point to solid circles which represent the autapses. All synapses represented by circles are "punctiform"; those represented by the "elongated" circles are "climbing fiber" arrangements, one of which is an autapse on dendrite 4. The caliber of the neuron's processes is not depicted in the trace; neither are spines on dendrites, nor small beads on axons. [Van der Loos and Glaser, 1972]

functions of these autapses. Van der Loos speculated that such a contact—arbitrarily assuming that it is inhibitory—may well be the substrate of a significant gating that puts part of the neuron's inputs under the control of the cell's own output. According to this hypothesis, excitatory synaptic inputs from other cells on the dendritic segment distal to an autapse would have their influence at the neuron's impulse-generating zone diminished by that autapse. Two assumptions underlie this hypothesis: (1) basal dendrites of neocortical pyramids conduct only passively, and (2) autapses are inhibitory. According to Rall (1970a), dendritic synaptic excitation is especially vulnerable to synaptic inhibition of the same dendritic location.

Gap Junction Ultrastructure: M. V. L. Bennett

Our knowledge of connectivity between cells, a matter most critical to the understanding of discrete versus continuous domain, has been extended by Bennett (1966, 1972a,b). From an electron micrographic reconstruction (see Figure 38), he presented a view of the gap junction as a sieve providing electrical and a small ion continuity (permeability established for Na^+, K^+, Cl^-, I^-, SO_4^{2-}, various dyes, and the molecule sucrose) between cells, while, at the same time, maintaining discontinuity for organelles.

A lattice made up of hexagons in the junction is obtained with lanthanum staining (among other treatments) and is interpreted as a set

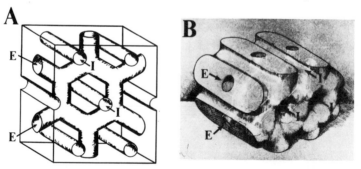

Figure 38. Proposed structure of gap junctions, diagrammatic (A) and less diagrammatic views (B). The arrows labeled E indicate the channels within the gap continuous with extracellular space. The arrows labeled I indicate the cytoplasmic channels running between cells in the bridges crossing the gap. The cytoplasmic faces are parallel to the plane of the page in A and to the lower right and back left in B. The overall thickness measured from cytoplasm to cytoplasm is about 150 A. The center-to-center spacing of the I channels is about 100 A. [Payton et al., 1969; Pappas et al., 1971]

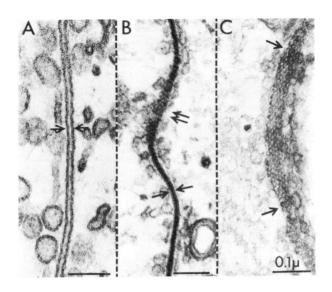

Figure 39. Electron micrographs of electrotonic synapses at septa of the crayfish septate axon. A. A thin section perpendicular to the closely apposed membranes. The overall thickness of the junction is about 180 A at the arrows. There is a central light area between the two unit membranes which is 30-40 A wide. B. Similar to A but the extracellular space between membranes is filled with a dense deposit of lanthanum that was present during fixation (Revel and Karnovsky, 1967). The overall thickness of the junction is about 165 A at the arrows. At the double arrow the membranes are cut somewhat tangentially and the lanthanum deposit appears not to be a uniform sheet. C. An approximately tangential section through the synaptic region following fixation in the presence of lanthanum. The lanthanum deposit (between arrows) forms a roughly hexagonal network outlining an array of clear regions. [Pappas et al., 1971]

of channels open to the extracellular space but closed to the intracellular space. Intracellular continuity can be demonstrated by the use of Procion yellow dye (Payton et al., 1969). Thus, these data suggest that the gap junction is made up of interlaced extracellular and intracellular channels (see Figure 39). Since the protein and lipid composition of isolated junctions has been shown to be quite simple, in agreement with EM and X-ray diffraction studies, further structural analysis at the molecular level can be expected (Goodenough and Stoeckenius, 1972).

According to Bennett, gap junctions are of widespread occurrence; they are found in mammalian CNS, retina, many epithelia such as liver, and cardiac and smooth muscle. Moreover, various cells in tissue culture can become coupled in minutes. As a reasonable hypothesis, he proposed that gap junctions are made by the union of preformed half-channels. The half-channels from one cell connect to the half-channels of an apposed cell and the resulting complete channels form a hexagonal array.

In Bennett's view, one function of this kind of junction is to maintain an electrotonic average of a group of cells, particularly those which fire synchronously, as in pacemaker nuclei controlling the electric organs of the electric catfish and *Gymnotus*. In the electric catfish, only two cells control the organ and they are strongly coupled; an impulse arising in either cell will always excite the other one and thus synchrony is assured. In *Gymnotus* the pacemaker cells are loosely coupled and impulses do not propagate from cell to cell unless the cells are very near their firing level. Because the cells are pacemaking at about the same frequency, even the weak coupling enables the earliest firing cell or cells to excite their neighbors, which are near threshold for firing, and thus all the cells fire nearly simultaneously. Although electrotonic coupling from one cell to another is weak, the summation of many such elements produces a strong effect. Trying experimentally to prevent one cell of the group from firing by hyperpolarizing is difficult; the individual cell continues to respond with group action. This is an example of an individual cell's function being determined by the group as contrasted with the group's function being determined by any strong activity of an individual cell. In this particular case, the principle of summation is obviously the most parsimonious one. It may be especially applicable under conditions of close synchronization, but in more complex systems, particularly in nonlinear couplings, this principle may not apply.

Relation of Synaptic to Electrotonic Influence

In the preceding examples, the coupling resistance presumably is purely a function of the area of a gap junction (or the number of such channels), and some rather nonquantitative correlation is available between the junctional area and resistance. It also turns out that neurons can be coupled by way of direct dendrodendritic and soma-somatic junctions or by way of presynaptic fibers ending on two or more cells.

The next two examples indicate that different inputs, including electrotonic ones, can be localized to different regions of the cell and thereby offer greater functional flexibility. Oculomotor neurons govern smoothly graded movements of the eyes, as well as sudden, stepwise movements such as the fast phase of nystagmus and eye withdrawal (Korn and Bennett, 1971). The control of two classes of movement by the same neurons requires more sophisticated regulation than the all-or-none synchronous electrical pulsing of electric fish. The oculomotor neurons as studied in fish by Bennett and his colleagues (see Kriebel et al., 1969; Korn and Bennett, 1972) are electrotonically coupled in the region of the cell bodies, but apparently not in dendritic regions. Impulses for sudden movements are produced by depolarizing postsynaptic potentials (PSP's) in the cell bodies, and the coupling mediates some increase in synchronization. Impulses for smoothly graded movements arise in the dendrites where there is no electrotonic interaction between excited neurons. Electrotonic separation of somatic and dendritic sites of impulse initiation is sufficiently great that no significant spread of PSP's takes place between them. The coupling between cell bodies is sufficiently weak that impulses do not propagate from cell to cell by way of the electrotonic pathway unless the postsynaptic cells are already depolarized by other inputs. Thus, impulses arising in the dendrites can propagate through the cell bodies without interacting.

In the opisthobranch mollusc *Navanax,* motoneurons in the buccal ganglia control both synchronous pharyngeal expansion for prey capture and asynchronous expansion for peristalsis (Spira and Bennett, 1972b). The motoneurons are electrotonically coupled during the first kind of movement and decoupled by synaptic inputs during the second kind of movement. The evidence suggests that the cells are functionally decoupled by inhibitory inputs localized along the pathway coupling them electrotonically. There is no evidence that the resistance of the gap junctions themselves is changed, although this remains a theoretical possibility.

Thus, Bennett finds that (1) electrotonically coupled neurons may act as one neuron or relatively independently, depending on the degree of coupling, and that (2) the degree of interaction can be regulated by locating excitatory inputs and coupling synapses on specific parts of the cell (see Figure 40) or by changing inhibitory inputs.

This evidence is a clear example of the progress made by regarding neural elements as simply summating to an aggregate property (further studies are being conducted by using classical neurophysiological concepts). It also elicits the question whether the more complex conceptualization centered around dynamic patterns is needed. Additionally, these findings are of great interest in establishing the concept of electrotonic cellular interaction leading to aggregate activity complementing the conventional synaptic one. A possible

MEDIAL RECTUS MOTONEURONS

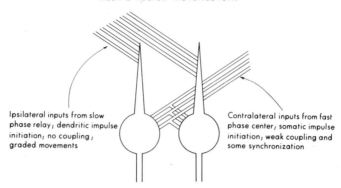

Ipsilateral inputs from slow
phase relay; dendritic impulse
initiation; no coupling;
graded movements

Contralateral inputs from fast
phase center; somatic impulse
initiation; weak coupling and
some synchronization

Figure 40. Diagram of oculomotor neurons. The cell bodies are coupled by way of presynaptic fibers. The dendrites are not coupled. [Korn and Bennett]

extrapolation in terms of this Work Session is that sustained aggregate activity of this kind would lead to the development of neural systems or "wholes" having modes of operation indicative of continuity, in addition to the conventional cellular discreteness underlying the synaptically coupled systems. Such electrotonic coupling may be critical in a learning model such as that of John (1972) in which the acquired reorganizing is based on the timing of many elements acting as an ensemble rather than on specific spatial connectivity changes. These electrotonic couplings may also contribute to a neural origin of some steady potential shifts (see below).

Macrostates, the Parts-Wholes Problem, and Fields: V. Rowland

A "macrostate variable," e.g., a variable that comprises the number of excitatory and inhibitory neurons firing at time t, is necessary for describing the nervous system on thermodynamic principles. The Wilson and Cowan model emphasizes the need to have an experimental equivalent of the macrostate. The intersections of the two curves (Figure 31B) in their phase plane, or the single intersection in the case of the limit cycle, indicates steady-state points of the macrostate for which response to perturbations has interesting specific characteristics. The macrostate is a theoretical construct, borrowed from thermodynamics, to which various physiological variables now in use may be compared and possibly better understood. Candidate variables are the massed neuronal firing record, the oscillatory field potentials (EEG), the steady or sustained potential field with its shifts (SPS), the available oxygen record, or even the millidegree temperature pattern. All these may contribute various pattern characteristics to the calculated theoretical macrostate dynamics.

One may anticipate other candidates for this macrostate measure and continue to speculate on the extent to which macrostate information is produced and utilized by the brain. It is presumed that it would be a measure of a holistic operation and its use might ultimately relate to the matrix of relations cybernetically modeled by Lange (1965).

We do not know to what degree a representation of the operation of all elements would be sensitive to qualitative or pattern changes within the totality of elements. It is quite likely that a macrostate representation of visual cortex would be insensitive in proportion to its size and duration; thus, a progressive subdivision would be necessary to enable detection of the difference in visual cortical processing, for example, between different visual patterns presented with equivalent luminous flux and an equivalent context in terms of subject interest. Recurrent subdivision, of course, leads to the concept of the microstate.

Wilson and Cowan specify that they require a high degree of redundancy in neural response in order to obtain a general dimension. It is noteworthy that the redundancy concept applied to nervous systems is challenged or qualified to one of extensive overlap or partial redundancy, especially for "higher nervous system" functions in the propositions of Bullock (1974).

One view of this dilemma is that neurons, when they lead to a type of behavioral response classed as generalizing by the experimenter, may be acting in a relatively redundant way, even though the information needed for less redundancy is present in their midst. On this basis, only when the total system's response is put into the service of discriminative behavior (when generalizations, so to speak, are broken up) will individual responses of elements show less redundancy.

Specifying spatial dimensions for a brain macrostate is too dependent on relative conditions to have much meaning. Nevertheless, if a 50 to 200 μ electrode detects the electrical contributions of hundreds or thousands of action potential generators located within a 1-mm diameter sphere, while at the same time detecting electrical fields having slower oscillations and shifts in a steady or sustained potential, detectable in the same locus, one may tentatively assign a relative macrostate character to these dependent variables for the purposes of interrelating them and setting up further observations.

The remarkable thing about this technique is that, although it would appear to be a wholesale smearing of all the incredibly elaborated microdetail and connectionism classically established in the nervous system, it does not yield up white noise or featureless records. Rather, temporal patterning of great detail is found; this means that all the microplusses and microminusses are not simply summated as if randomly distributed in time and space. (By contrast, if one places two small wire ends in Ringer's solution and differentially amplifies the irregular contact potentials arising from each, one records many large, random, voltage fluctuations. If the exposed wire surface is now progressively enlarged, the fluctuations are progressively summed, cancel each other at arriving at an average, and eventually disappear altogether.)

The question then arises whether the patterning seen with probes that transgress boundaries conventionally taken to define the discreteness, as opposed to the continuity of the systems under observation, can inform us of system properties essential to the overall operation. In this sense, the patterns are space-time macrostates by which we may ultimately come to understand the qualities of the whole system.

A full description of the system depends on both the matrix of element relations and the matrix of element properties according to Lange (1965).* The contemporary view of the oscillatory and steady potential fields gives the experimenter information about the system essential for an understanding of element participation (see Freeman, below). The notion that the fields, themselves, produce information affecting system function is still controversial, but indirect evidence for that view arose at the Work Session (see the discussions of Adey above and Morrell below).

We cannot now make a clear distinction between undemarcated system properties (e.g., EEG and SPS) and similar vague macrostates. For the moment, we rest with their crude comparison on the basis of their not only informing us about totalities emerging from seemingly

---

*Katchalsky referred repeatedly to this work of the Polish cyberneticist, Oskar Lange, which, unfortunately, is no longer in print in English. Katchalsky was much impressed with Lange's matrix algebra representation of complex systems and with his analysis of the emergence of "properties of the whole" relying on at least two sets of variables—those describing the element properties and those describing the relations of the elements.

infinite complexity, but also providing us with organizing information about elements not obtainable from the elements themselves.

Oscillating Fields and Pulse Distributions

Relation of Neuronal Waves to EEG: R. Elul

Elul has reversed his thinking about the low coherence between the electrical oscillations inside the neuron ("neuronal waves") and the much lower voltage oscillogram ("gross EEG") recorded outside the cell or on the brain surface (Figure 41). Formerly, he viewed this as an absence of a relationship or coupling and saw the low incidence of coinciding oscillographic pattern in the element and the aggregate as mere chance coincidence. By blocking action potential conduction with tetrodotoxin as a means of brief functional disconnection (Figures 42 and 43), he found evidence of thalamocortical timing of silent periods, which led him to view the momentary episodes of coherence between the element and gross pattern as a period of coupling. All incoherent periods are now seen as periods of nonparticipation of the element with the aggregate that intervenes between brief periods of participation. The oscillograms, whether intra- or extraneuronally recorded, are viewed as patterns of postsynaptic potentials arising from many

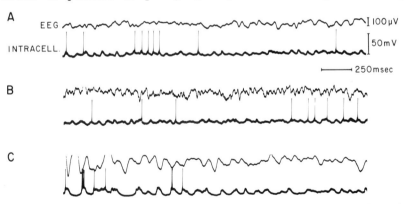

Figure 41. Neuronal wave activity recorded with intracellular microelectrode. Animal is awake in A, sleeping in B, and intensely aroused in C, with EEG patterns characteristic of each of these states. Note the corresponding changes in the form of the neuronal waves. A to C are from same cell in posterior suprasylvian cortex, 750 μ in depth; micropipette filled with KCl solution. EEG taken from anterior suprasylvian cortex on contralateral hemisphere. [Elul, 1968]

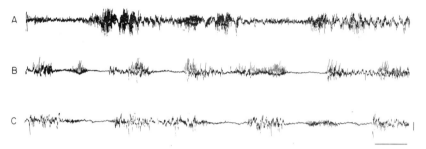

Figure 42. Effect of intraventricular tetrodotoxin on EEG. A. Taken just before injection of the drug. B. 10 min later. C. 20 min following the injection. Bipolar recording from surface electrodes making contact with the dura (parietal-parietal). Calibration: 1 sec, 50 μV. [Elul, 1972a]

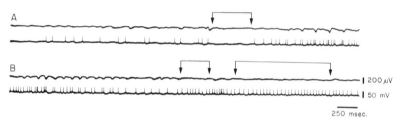

Figure 43. Effect of tetrodotoxin on neuronal wave activity and on EEG. Unanesthetized cat, 950-μ depth in sigmoid cortex; EEG taken from surface about 1.5 mm away. A and B. Successive episodes of EEG "flattening" (delimited by arrows). Note inconsistent behavior of nerve cell during three episodes. [Elul, 1972a]

thousands of synaptic connections. The amplitudes of these oscillations vary directly as the number of generators operating *synchronously,* whereas signals arising from *nonsynchronized* generators increase only as the square root of the number of generators. Elul (1972a,b) postulates that, in all likelihood, nonsynchronized generators could not produce a sufficient voltage to be seen by contemporary techniques. Thus, all activity visible in the EEG spectrum relates to some degree of synchrony. On the basis of cortex undercutting and the tetrodotoxin experiments, Elul concludes that the thalamus is scanning the cortex. (See the scanning concept of Pitts and McCulloch, 1947.) The implication is that the EEG *frequency* reflects the scanning *frequency* and the EEG *amplitude* reflects the ensemble *size* (number of synchronized participating generators). Even if the processes should not turn out to be scanning, but rather a sequencing of ensembles developing with less dependence on fixed dominant pacemakers, the model relates to the temporal organizing model of John (1972) and the phase-relation model of Freeman (see below).

Dynamic Pattern in Sequencing and Synchrony

In relation to dynamic patterns, the sequencing rate described above can be viewed as being determined either by the cooperative activity of a number of elements operating in a limit-cycle mode or by the fixed connectivity of a set of pacemakers. The resolution of this question in the direction of a group determination of frequency and amplitude rather than a pacemaker determination would emphasize the utility of dynamic pattern theory in understanding multineuronal systems.

Elul's mathematical model for the dynamics of neural populations is based on the work of Anninos and his co-workers (1970; Anninos, 1972b). Anninos investigated the behavior of a discrete population of 1000 "formal" neurons with fixed geometry by means of computer simulation (Figure 44). The neural populations were specified by a number of parameters: fraction of inhibitory neurons, average number of connections to each cell, the firing threshold of the neurons, and synaptic delay. Time (n) is an integral multiple of the synaptic delay. Figure 44 shows the distributions of firing neurons at various times defined by Anninos and his co-workers (1970) as the state vector a_n of the neural population. Figure 44A shows that, at times 9 and 31, the state vectors are different although both states have the same total number of active neurons. After a time lapse of 76 synaptic delays, a cyclic pattern develops: $a_{76} = a_{82} = a_{88}$ (Figure 44B) and no new states will appear ($a_{77} = a_{83} = a_{89} \ldots$). The successive new states a_{77}, a_{78}, and a_{79} are, however, different (Figure 44C).

Elul's model is like a multiplexing system—the thalamus scanning the cortex periodically. A major difference is that the scan may not rigidly sample a given locus at a systematic interval nor all loci at a fixed sequencing rate. It is conceivable that the multiplexing system is of a nonspecific origin modulated by activity impinging at both thalamus and cortex. The system would influence the rate of scan and dwell time at preferred loci, especially those regions mediating ongoing inputs. The EEG amplitudes may reflect the size of the synchronized ensemble participating in the content of perception at any given moment, and the EEG frequencies may reflect the rapidity with which the sequencing of ensembles occurs.

The meaning of reduced amplitude and increased frequency of the EEG ("activation") is, then, a spatial constriction of overall (cortex and thalamus) ensemble size in order that a more localized (and smaller) subset may be sequenced more frequently. Increased temporal

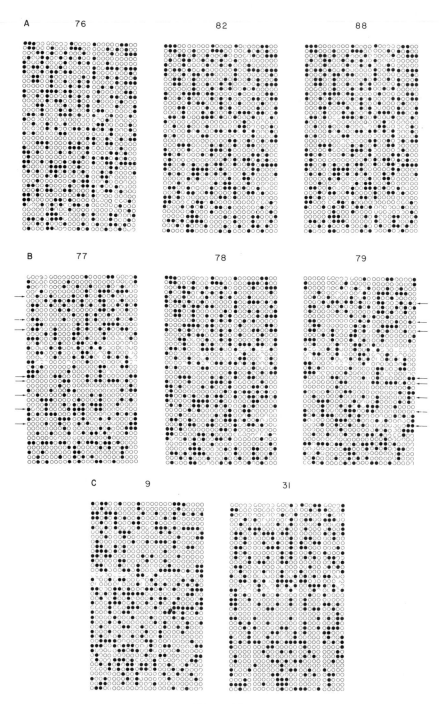

Figure 44

resolution is obtained by restricting overall nonspecific connectivity. When the environment makes no demands on the organism, its brain can "idle," its scans now encompassing a spatially expanded or more distributed number of elements but sequencing at a slower rate. One can artificially stimulate such a system as in recruitment (the successive incrementing of wave amplitudes with stimulus repetition in the 3 to 12 Hz range) and evoke coherent wave activity from a variety of loci, all of them equivalent entries into a synchronizable system. The synchronizability would then be a function of the system rather than of any subset of elements within it. The system is more dependent on stimulus frequency than stimulus locus, the slower frequencies being capable of synchronizing larger or more distributed aggregates.

If the mechanism controlling the locus of synchronizing influence turns out to be a continuously shifting one, two basic possibilities arise. The shifting may be rigidly determined by intrinsically fixed connectivity, i.e., anatomically determined, in which case a mechanism based on dynamic pattern theory would not be likely. Alternatively, it may represent the activity of loosely coupled loci of influence, moving unpredictably or statistically through different neuronal populations but providing, in the mass (macrostate), either a dynamic pattern with stable regions and "jump" transitions or limit-cycle activity.

The flow pattern (EEG) would not depend on tight and possibly quite redundant coupling of the element (neuron) dynamics simply summed, but on statistical system characteristics of large groups of elements. No element will exhibit a contributory pattern except in such an evanescent way as to be scarcely differentiable from chance coincidence.

Figure 44. Firing patterns in artificial nerve nets. All diagrams drawn from the same nerve net and represent activity at different points in time, as indicated at the top of each diagram. Solid and open circles indicate active and inactive neurons, respectively. A. The three state vectors at times n = 76, 82, and 88 are identical; these represent recycling of the same firing pattern. B. Activity in the intervening periods assumes a different pattern: the three consecutive state vectors (n = 77, 78, 79) are inside the cycle from 76 to 82 in A, and they differ among themselves and also from the state vector of n = 76 or 82 (although the diagrams of n = 77 and 79 appear similar, they differ in a number of points indicated by the arrows). The number of firing neurons does not determine the state vector at the same time. C. Shows two state vectors (n = 9, 31) with identical number of firing neurons, but the distribution of these neurons in the net, as indicated by the corresponding state vectors illustrated here, is rather different. Net parameters for A to C are as follows: number of neurons = 1,000; minimal number of excitatory postsynaptic potentials needed to trigger a neuron in the absence of inhibitory postsynaptic potentials = 1; average number of axon branches emanating from each neuron = 4; and fraction of inhibitory neurons = 40% of the total population, i.e., 400. [Adapted from Anninos, 1972a]

Pulse-Wave Problems: W. J. Freeman

Freeman (1972a,b,c,d,e,f,g) reviewed pulse (action potential)-wave (EEG) relations as developed in his extensive studies on the olfactory bulb and related structures. By suggesting terms newly and carefully defined (aggregates, populations, cartels, and systems), he provided both a semantics and a set of concepts that enable a simultaneous consideration of system properties and element functions. At the Work Session, Freeman confirmed the utility of recognizing that the neural masses in the central nervous system maintain innumerable nonlinear interactions that preclude reduction by simple summation. Emphasizing that true interactions must be carefully discriminated from coincidental and co-driven actions, he thinks that the dynamic pattern model offers much needed sets of testable equations for predicting the properties of cell systems and a promising direction for future research on this very difficult problem.

The application of the theory of nonequilibrium processes to the nervous system is based on two equivalences. The time-dependent responses of sets of neurons play the role of chemical reactions, and the transmission of neural activity by axons and dendrites through synapses is equivalent to diffusion. Spatially and temporally continuous dynamic patterns ("dissipative structures") arise in a set of neurons only if they are functionally interconnected at high density. If anatomical feedback connections do not exist among a set of neurons, or if the function of the connections is suppressed by anesthesia, the function of the set approaches an equilibrium state. If feedback through dense synaptic complexes is strong enough, the set of neurons goes through one or more state transitions to reach a nonequilibrium steady state in which complex spatiotemporal patterns of neural activity occur.

Analysis of the function of interactive sets is facilitated by the description of a hierarchy of topologies of connection. This concept was developed by Freeman in an analysis of the vertebrate olfactory system (Figure 45). At the lowest level of the hierarchy is the "aggregate," formed, for example, by the olfactory receptors, R. These have no anatomical synaptic interconnections and are shown schematically as a single circle in Figure 46. The lowest interactive level is the "population," which arises from interaction among neurons that are either all excitatory or all inhibitory. Five examples are shown in Figures 45 and 46 as pairs of circles linked by double arrows having plus (+) or minus (−) signs to signify mutual excitation or mutual

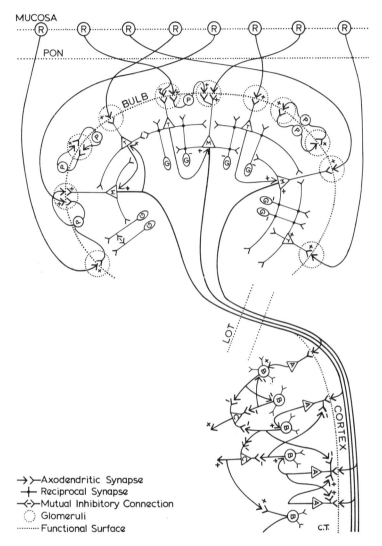

Figure 45. This is a diagram of the neuron types of the olfactory system and their connections. All types of connections and feedback loops are shown. The levels of neural mass (aggregate, population, cartel, and system) are based on these connection types. Although each schematic neuron is shown making a few connections, each neuron in the bulb and cortex makes the indicated types of connection innumerable times. + = excitation; – = inhibition; A = type A neuron (superficial pyramidal cell); B = type B neuron (short axon or cortical granule cell); C = type C neuron (deep pyramidal cell); G = granule cell; LOT = lateral olfactory tract; M,T = mitral, tufted neuron; P = periglomerular neuron; PON = primary olfactory nerve; R = olfactory receptor. [Freeman, 1972g]

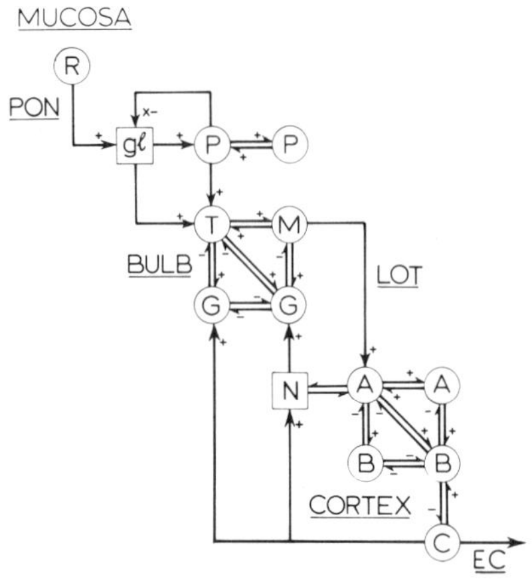

Figure 46. This is a lumped-circuit diagram showing the main functional connections within the two olfactory complex cartels located in the bulb and cortex and the polarities of connection. + = excitation; − = inhibition; x− = multiplicative inhibition (related to presynaptic inhibition); EC = external capsule; gl = glomeruli; N = anterior olfactory nucleus; for other abbreviations, see legend to Figure 45. [Freeman, 1973b]

inhibition. Populations have only positive feedback and give prolonged nonoscillatory responses on single shock electrical stimulation (Knight, 1972; Freeman, 1973c).

The interaction of an excitatory population with an inhibitory population gives rise to a more complex interactive mass called a "cartel," which is capable of oscillatory behavior on impulse stimulation. It has negative feedback in addition to the two kinds of positive feedback. This concept is at the level of the model developed by Wilson and Cowan (1972). One cartel exists in the olfactory bulb and one in the prepiriform cortex (Figures 45 and 46), and Freeman proposed that these two interactive masses provide the neural bases for the bulbar and cortical EEG's and oscillatory averaged evoked potentials (AEP's).

The concatenation of aggregates, populations, and cartels, as in Figures 45 and 46, forms a neural "system" that corresponds to the level of function assigned to parts of the brain which are identified as specific sensory or motor systems. The hierarchy serves as a conceptual bridge between the functional properties of single neurons and the holistic properties of the set of neurons comprising a sensory or motor channel.

The essence of this view is that the collective properties of the set cannot be predicted from or reduced to the properties of the component neurons. Observation and measurement must be directed to events occurring at the level of the interactive mass. Unitary events at the level of a single neuron can then be interpreted in relation to the properties of either the neuron and its parts or the mass, of which the neuron is a part. This is why Freeman attaches great importance to measurements of AEP's and EEG's, which are direct manifestations of massive neural interactions.

As an example of an interactive property, Freeman described a statistical analysis of the spike train of a single mitral cell (M in Figures 45 and 46) in relation to the EEG field potential concomitantly generated by granule cells (G in Figures 45 and 46), both neuron types being members of the same bulbar cartel. The reciprocal dendro-dendritic synaptic interconnections are excitatory (mitral to granule) and inhibitory (granule to mitral) and form a negative feedback loop (Rall and Shepherd, 1968). The characteristic output for such a loop is predicted to be an oscillation at about 40 Hz (Freeman, 1972c), and this prediction is confirmed for the granule cells by spectral analysis of the bulbar EEG. However, the autocovariance of the mitral pulse train shows no sign of periodicity (Figure 47A).

In contrast, the probability of pulse occurrence conditional on the amplitude of the EEG (Freeman, 1972a) does show periodicity (Figure 47B). The comparison shows that, if the pulse train is interpreted with respect to the properties of the single neuron, it appears to resemble a random pulse train. If it is analyzed with respect to the properties of the neural mass (the EEG), it manifests oscillation in pulse probability at the frequency of the ensemble. The oscillation, which is called a pulse probability wave (Freeman, 1972g), has a particular phase that can only be measured with respect to the ensemble mean manifested in the EEG of the interactive mass.

In Freeman's view, the EEG is not part of the mechanism. The extracellular fields of current have neither the geometry nor the local intensity to influence significantly the performance of bulbar and cortical neurons. A synaptic field of activity (a "dissipative structure") gives rise to a field of synaptic current, but the current field is neither necessary nor sufficient to establish the synaptic field. The EEG is merely an electrical epiphenomenon that permits observation of events in the mass.

The problem of stationarity of the phase relation of the mitral or tufted cell's firing with the 40 Hz burst pattern of the EEG relates to anesthesia and its level. In the unanesthetized animal, stationarity cannot be maintained for more than 5 to 10 sec according to Freeman,

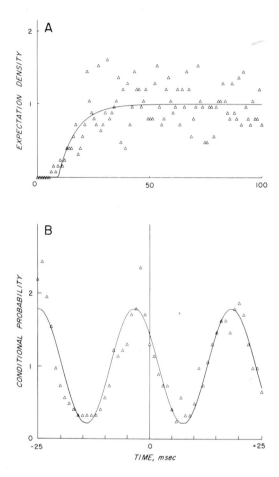

Figure 47. A. Shows the expectation density computed from the pulse train of a single mitral-tufted cell during spontaneous or background activity. The absolute and relative refractory periods are seen, but there is no oscillation in pulse probability with post-pulse time. B. Shows (for the same pulse train) the conditional pulse probability as a function of time on EEG amplitudes from +1 to +3 standard deviations from the mean amplitude of zero. The oscillation in pulse probability is at the frequency of the EEG. Both probability functions are normalized by dividing the values by the mean pulse probability. The oscillation (B) is a pulse probability curve. It is a property of the active mass of neurons and not of the single neuron. [Freeman, 1972g]

unless behavior is very carefully controlled. In lightly anesthetized animals, with careful control of stimulation, stationarity can be extended up to one-half hour, and, in deep anesthesia, extended even further. An appropriate question is whether the well-appreciated desynchronizing tendency of the waking state imposes a severe constraint on the observability of these relations. Furthermore,

Freeman does not generalize these observations to sensory systems other than the olfactory and believes that the analysis may require 250,000 action potentials obtained over a 4-min sampling period.

Postsynaptic Events: W. A. Spencer

With intracellular recordings, Spencer and his colleagues (Spencer and Kandel, 1961c; Kandel et al., 1961; Gessi, 1971; Lebovitz et al., 1971) have used antidromic activation of hippocampal pyramidal cells in the deafferented fornix preparation to evoke dynamic neuronal patterns and field potentials that, in their view, may be explained without invoking nonsynaptic electrical or chemical interactions as mediating agencies (Figure 48). They have demonstrated an inhibitory postsynaptic potential (IPSP) using intracellular recordings that can last 10 times longer than the 10- to 20-msec wave transient recorded extracellularly as a field event. The latter appears at the onset of the prolonged IPSP and has been interpreted to indicate that basket-type

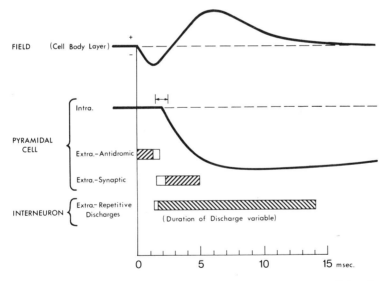

Figure 48. Summary diagram of time relations of responses of different cellular elements following single shock to deafferented fornix. Hatched portions of bars indicate periods of greatest firing probability; clear zones are periods of infrequent firing. This diagram presents the usual time relations encountered. It should be noted that transynaptically evoked pyramidal cell responses to stimulation of the deafferented fornix (Extra.-Synaptic) indicate the operation of recurrent excitatory pathways. The intracellularly recorded IPSP (Intra.) indicates recurrent inhibitory actions. These systems provide positive and negative feedback, respectively. [Lebovitz et al., 1971]

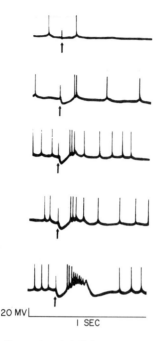

Figure 49. Responses to stimulation of the deafferented fornix at progressively increasing stimulus intensities. Note the appearance of recurrent inhibition followed by late excitation with repetitive firing. [Spencer and Kandel, 1961c]

20 MV

I SEC

cells mediate the inhibition (Andersen et al., 1964). The disparity in time course can be attributed only partially to the rather long time constant of these pyramidal neurons (Spencer and Kandel, 1961a). However, with low-stimulus currents (1.2 times threshold), the field potential was found to be much more enduring and to come into closer agreement with the IPSP time course (Gessi, 1971). Stronger stimuli evidently bring in other actions that produce the characteristic composite field potential of short duration. Long-enduring recurrent IPSP's are observed from all parts of the hippocampus and thus appear to be a general characteristic of the pyramidal neurons. Even the late phases of this recurrent inhibition may be produced by the rich terminal plexus of the basket-type cells in the pyramidal cell layer, since the slower field potential also has a depth configuration which shows an inflection at or near the level of pyramidal cell bodies.

This prolonged recurrent IPSP of hippocampal neurons can generate rebound excitation very similar to that described by Andersen and Eccles (1962) for ventrobasal thalamic neurons. It may thus induce rebound oscillation for 1 or 2 cycles (Spencer and Kandel, 1961c) alternating with brief excitatory phases in an overall pattern that appears as a damped oscillation (Figure 49). These rebound phenomena may be rather complex because of involvement of more circuitous paths. Still, Spencer sees these approaches based on defining connectionist interactions between excitatory and inhibitory recurrent pathways as potentially sufficient for the more complete analysis of oscillatory phenomena (Andersen and Andersson, 1968). It seems unnecessary to invoke field interactions of a nonsynaptic nature to explain such kinds of oscillation. Nonsynaptic mechanisms may be important, however, in the genesis of hippocampal seizures (Dichter et al., 1972), as discussed below (see "Pathologic Dynamic Patterns").

Steady States and Their Shifts: V. Rowland

The more we learn about the properties of EEG, the more ambiguous the term becomes, since, for some investigators, it refers only to scalp-recorded activity in contrast to the electrocorticogram (ECoG). It may include for some researchers, and exclude for others, the base-line changes now well established in the literature on steady and sustained potential shifts (SPS) and on the contingent negative variation (CNV). In some contexts, it is also the extracellular pattern recorded by macroelectrodes (e.g., Elul's "gross EEG") and used in differentiation from the very similar, but usually noncoherent, pattern inside the cell called neuronal waves. In some contexts, further problems arise from consideration of the EEG as relatively slow-wave activity (in contrast to fast "spiky" activity) when "slow" and "fast" frequencies occur within the EEG (Perkel and Bullock, 1968).* Whatever course comes to prevail semantically, it now appears that there is an essential distinction between oscillatory and nonoscillatory electrical field dynamics. This fundamental difference in pattern, now investigated in terms of precise identification of the generators, also points to a fundamental difference in system properties or "qualities of the whole." The reason this difference has escaped attention is because only recently have we acquired enough information about a nonoscillatory potential pattern to discern that the fundamental distinguishing

---

*On the basis of the above, the Table of "Forms of Representation of Information in the Nervous System" presented in the "Appendix" of Perkel and Bullock (1968) should be amended as follows: The title for item 2 in "III. Ensemble Activity, C. Representation by Form of Composite of Multiunit Activity. 2. Slow waves in ongoing EEG" should become "Electric oscillations in brain tissue." A new item "Steady or sustained potentials and their shifts" should be added as item 3. The reader may develop for himself, from the relevant information below, the facts as far as they go for entries under "referent," "transformation," "transmission," and "interpretation." Consideration should also be given to the neuronal waves of Elul as either a subdivision of IA 5: "Membrane potential: spatial and temporal distribution," or as a new entry IA 6: "Intraneuronal electric oscillation." See the discussions of Spencer and Grossman for the possibility of a further entry: "Intraneuronal nonoscillatory patterns."

feature of the conventional EEG is not that it is electrical (the theory that it is an active modulating influence as an electrical field is challenged by many investigators) or encephalic (found in many different regions of the brain and not in the spinal cord), but rather that it is an oscillatory system. That this pattern can "ride" on a base line that shifts in a nonoscillatory manner (SPS) is a fact not generally included in the connotations of the term EEG. Whether SPS should be included or excluded in the formal definition of EEG is much less important than developing a better understanding of the nature and degree of coupling, if any, between the oscillating and nonoscillating systems observed by use of electrical potentials. It is suggested that we could make semantic progress commensurate with our experiments by dropping the term EEG and substituting oscillogram, using whatever adjectives are needed for labeling its origin (e.g., "intracellular," "bulk tissue," "gross"). Either "steady" or "sustained" potentials with their shifts are the terms proposed for the electrical nonoscillatory patterns observed in brain tissue or the spinal cord. Because the reactivity of SPS strongly suggests a system property in its own right, and not just the absence of oscillation, it would be most helpful if a more specific functional name could be applied to it at the present time. However, the origins and underlying actions for steady-state changes in the brain as recorded electrically are not yet well enough understood to justify this. Freeman suggests that a bias function is the central defining feature reflected by SPS, but this has yet to be established unequivocally, since Rowland has observed in "quiet expectancy" an SPS unattended by action potential changes (see Figures 53 and 54 below).

To the extent steady-state systems are causatively coupled with oscillatory systems or numerous generators of fast transients, they must operate in some way as a determinant of, or constraint on, the dynamics of the oscillators. This relation must be distinguished from by-product or epiphenomenal steady states that arise in a system by the unspecific summation of many element variables. If this summation yields a time integral that cannot be demonstrated to affect the elements that produce it, it may not operate as a system constraint but may still yield information as a macrostate indicator of the changes in the average over many contributors. In this sense, the roles are reversed, the oscillators and transient generators are now a determinant of, or a constraint on, the steady state. The degree of coupling and the direction of the dependency between steady-state and oscillator systems may vary nonlinearly, and we can intuit all manner of possible complexities that may arise from these conditions.

Behavioral Studies

Two Types of Shift

The genesis of brain and spinal cord steady or sustained potential shifts and the nature and extent of their coupling with oscillating systems and action potential distributions are only modestly understood. In the cortex of behaving animals, Rowland has observed two kinds of SPS: SPS-1, which is stimulus-bound, and SPS-2, which varies with the associative and drive contexts into which the environmental stimulus is delivered. Because SPS-2 can be varied with the animal's habit strength (H, the associational context) and drive state (D, the reinforcement history), it has been tentatively compared with a hypothetical internal variable introduced by Hull, called reaction potential (E), the product of H and D (Rowland, 1968). Paraphrasing Hullian theory (Hull, 1952), an animal's performance, according to either a speed or an error criterion, is considered to depend on E, its potential to react. In a still broader sense, the behavioral optimization of a subject's performance depends on both its "willingness" (D) and "ability"(H).

SPS-1 is believed to be more directly related to the reception of environmental stimuli, responses of specific systems, and to specific motor acts. Figure 50 shows examples of SPS-1 with a striking correlation of an integration of massed unit activity obtained from the same electrodes as used for SPS recording. Mass unit activity is often found to produce integration curves correlated with SPS-1 in a manner similar to that seen with cortical transients: evoked responses, lambda waves, spontaneous high-voltage slow rhythms, and poststimulus "ringing." Rebert (1969, 1973) has shown similar effects in the lateral geniculate. Internal (midcortical) referencing in these SPS's enables demonstration of surface-positive, depth-negative mirroring in the visual cortex in the same manner as seen for evoked responses and other wave transients. The latter presumably relate to a spatial distribution of generators like that for a dipole pattern of radially oriented neurons with a current source at the cortical surface and a sink at the 4th cortical layer and below. However, a gradient of positivity decreasing from cortical surface to depth, or of negativity increasing toward the depth, can give the same result and is observed with other electrode combinations. The precise nature of this pattern has yet to be determined and may ultimately require consideration of dynamic patterns of the types described by Katchalsky in addition to simpler models of sources and sinks of current flow.

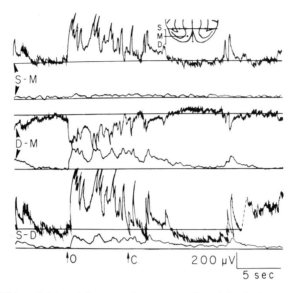

Figure 50. SPS-1 and integrated mass unit responses from left visual cortex of cat with orienting response induced by opening the cage door (arrow at O) and subsiding after closure (arrow at C). Implanted tripole with prefixed 0.5-mm separation of its tips was placed so that the surface (S), mid (M), and depth (D) layers of cortex were recorded. Upper tracing of each pair provides the oscillatory and SPS portion of the ECoG; lower, the integration of mass unit activity (IMU) derived from the same electrode pair providing the ECoG. Note that SPS was evoked with orienting and was associated with an increment in IMU. Prominent sharp waves are lambda waves associated with saccades. Time courses of SPS and IMU are similar except for a minimal or an absent change in the surface derivation of IMU. Calibration amplitude for 200 μV in ECoG also represents an increment of 20 μV in peak-to-peak amplitude of mass unit activity. Positivity is up in this and subsequent figures of this section. [Rowland]

SPS-1 has been observed in visual, auditory, and somesthetic cortex, but not sufficiently on a simultaneously recorded basis to determine the extent to which it is specific to the modality stimulated. Present data suggest a predominant shift in the cortical analyzer stimulated, but the cortical analyzers for other modalities also react to some extent with SPS, either as part of a less specific activation or as a sign of intersensory participation in response to a stimulus to the receptors of just one modality.

Trend to Graded Shifts with Experience

SPS-2 is distinguishable primarily by modifiability through reinforcement conditions that alter the subject's "reaction potential" (Hullian E) and by its lack of direct dependence on external stimulation. In lever-pressing rats placed on a fixed 1-min schedule of

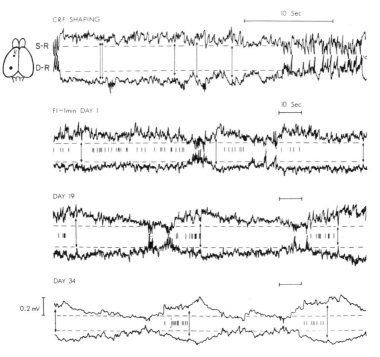

Figure 51. Acquisition of SPS-2 in a rat on a fixed 1-min schedule. Dot on brain diagram (*upper left*) is locus of vertically oriented electrode pair at cortical surface (S-R) and cortical depth (D-R) 1 mm subjacent. Referred against a cortical surface reference at R, S-R provides a symmetrically opposite voltage to that seen at D-R. CRF (continuous reinforcement) shaping schedule provides a pellet (arrow) for each lever press. No SPS pattern was present and an S−, D+ shift accompanies synchrony during inactive period. By Day 19 of a fixed 1-min training, rat acquires a stable SPS pattern (see the text). Lever presses (short vertical hatch marks) become grouped at the end of the interval and are often predicted by the reversal of SPS polarity. Day 34 sample was filtered to suppress conventional oscillogram and emphasize SPS. [Anderson]

reinforcement (Figure 51), Anderson* observed an acquisition of SPS-2 on the order of $200\,\mu V$, with an anticipatory surface-positive component and a cortical depth-negative component in the visual cortex. This shift is acquired with increasing regularity of pattern as the animal gains experience in the program. The pattern reverses direction shortly after the rat consumes its pellet reward, continuing until about the middle of the 1-min interval, and then again reverses direction some seconds before the animal resumes lever pressing. This pattern is not a passive concomitant of bar pressing, because animals on fixed-ratio (FR) schedules of 50 lever presses per reward show very similar steady potential shifts, even though they are lever pressing throughout the

*R. Anderson, unpublished data.

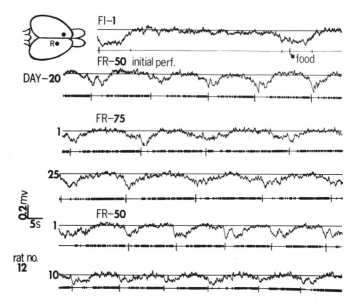

Figure 52. A. Effect of varying the ratio of lever presses to reinforcement on abruptness and gradation of SPS-2. Derivation has the left hemisphere stigmatic locus on brain surface at the dot, referred against the locus at R. Fixed 1-min schedule shows well-trained responses prior to switching to FR training. With a ratio of 50, rat acquired smooth arcs for which sample at Day 20 is shown. The first day of change to FR-75 is shown with "ledges" appearing towards the end of the intertrial interval in many trials at the time the animal showed retention of expectancy of reward at 50. Subsequently, as sampled on the 25th day after the change, smoother arcs were much more frequent and "ledges" were rare. When replaced on FR-50, the animal had abrupt shifts (arrow) with an unexpected appearance of the pellet on the first day (compare Day 20 of first training on FR-50). Subsequently, evidence of return to smoother arcs appears as shown in sample at Day 10. [Anderson]

intervals during which the SPS shows a clear reversal of direction. The direction of shift is independent of the act of lever pressing and appears more likely relatable to the animal's expectancy state, as revealed in the time course of the SPS throughout the interval between reinforcements.

Figure 52A shows shifts produced in relation to a fixed-ratio performance with smooth arcs generated to FR-50, disruption of the prereinforcement segment of these when the ratio is increased to 75 (prolongations or "ledges" developing just before reinforcement), but a return to more regular arcing with further experience on the new schedule. On return to the FR-50 schedule, the smooth arcs are distorted by abrupt shifts produced by the unexpected reinforcements. With further experience the subject develops a return of the smooth arcs. The SPS-2 pattern, therefore, appears to relate to an expectancy macrostate with the well-trained subject developing smooth gradients,

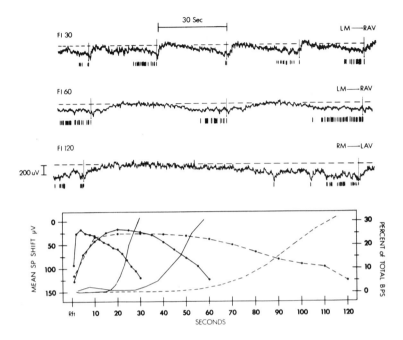

Figure 52. B. *Upper half,* patterns of SP shifting recorded during the fixed interval (FI) training with intervals of 30 sec (top), 1 min (middle), and 2 min (bottom). Records from three different rats. In each record, bar pressing is anticipated and accompanied by a sustained SP shift. Electrode placements are given at the right (LM-RAV = left motor with right anterior visual reference, RM-LAV = right motor with left anterior visual reference). Reinforced (arrows) and nonreinforced bar presses are shown as vertical marks below the corresponding record. *Lower half,* mean amplitude of shift (downward curving arcs) and percent of total bar presses (BPS, upward curving graphs) as a function of time during FI performance. Note the direct correspondence between the slope of the shift (activation) gradient and the distribution of bar presses with intersections of curves falling near a constant SPS voltage (about 50% of maximum) and percentage of bar presses (15%) for all three intervals. Number of subjects: 5 for FI 30-sec performance, 12 for FI 1-min performance, and 11 for FI 2-min performance. Data points were determined by averaging 120 reinforced intervals per rat. [Anderson]

the naive or recently rescheduled subject showing two kinds of departures from smooth gradation.

The slopes of these arcs in a fixed-interval program depend on the length of the interval (Figure 52B). The averaged curve of the steady potential shift, displayed with the curves of the relative bar presses for each interval, shows intersections occurring at the same level of SPS development for each schedule (about 75 μV). At this point each subject has emitted about 15% of his total lever presses for the interval. As can be seen in the record samples, the steady potential shifts clearly precede the onset of lever pressing.

Quiet Expectancy

Rowland observed similar anticipatory shifts in cat visual cortex under conditions of nonoperant training. The subject in Figure 53 was noncontingently given 5 ml of a milk-fish homogenate at 7-min intervals in the dark. Detection of the reinforcement was olfactory, the animal being trained to a constant position in a plastic cylinder with the food cup 2 cm from its nose. Simultaneous recording of SPS, the oscillogram, and integrated mass unit activity revealed that the animal acquired a temporally conditioned steady potential shift over the 2- to 3-min interval preceding reinforcements. There was no concomitant *sustained* elevation in the unit activity record. The latter was, however, responsive to transients related to saccades (the lambda wave activity), to conditioned clicks, to light flashes, and to motor and sensory activity accompanying consummatory response (licking).

In two loci, a very clear anticipatory steady potential shift, dissociated from sustained unit activity, was observed (Figure 52). The

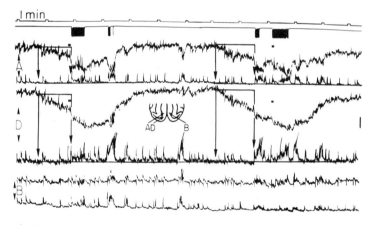

Figure 53. SPS-2 in "quiet expectancy" dissociated from sustained alteration of mass unit activity derived from same electrodes. Two cycles of characteristic record are shown. They were obtained after temporal conditioning was established by feeding 5 ml of a milk-fish homogenate every 7 min. Feeding occurs at time shown by small solid rectangle just before lickometer response registers in second channel. Individual lickometer deflections were compressed into a single mass. Brackets with arrows show 1- to 2-min interval of "quiet expectancy" with a sharp drop in SPS at loci A and D (recorded against a remote reference) and unattended by any sustained alteration in integration of mass unit activity (lower tracing of each pair used per locus). The latter can, however, show sustained increments at the time of obtaining food or other activity during restoration and waiting phases of intertrial interval. At site B, recorded against the same reference, an absence of a shift tends to exclude the reference as a source for a shift. Conspicuous transients in ECoG and integrated mass units records are, respectively, lambda waves and the associated unit activity with each wave. Voltage calibrations = 100 μV for ECoG, 10 μV for units. [Rowland]

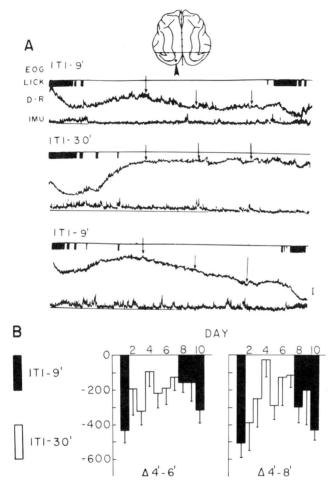

Figure 54. A. An expectancy shift (as in Figure 53) present for a 9-min temporal conditioning (intertrial interval, ITI, = 9) is lost after changing to a 30-min ITI for 5 days. After changing back to a 9-min ITI for 3 days, the expectancy shift is restored. D-R is point D of Figure 53 to a remote reference. IMU is an integration of multiple unit activity. Arrows show measurement times at 4, 6, and 8 min following the delivery of reinforcement and the beginning of licking. Note the absence of sustained IMU alteration during the prominent slope of expectancy SPS-2. Voltage calibrations are the same as those for Figure 53. EOG = electrooculogram. B. Means and standard errors of shift amplitudes obtained over 2-min ($\Delta 4'$-$6'$) and 4-min ($\Delta 4'$-$8'$) intervals between arrows shown in A. Amplitudes are measured from maximum positivity occurring after feeding. [Rowland]

third locus did not show this shift, and it was recorded against the same remote reference as the other loci. With further training, the animal retained an anticipatory shift with respect to a 9-min interval (Figure 54A). Over 6 days of experience with a 30-min interval (control for temporal conditioning of the 9-min interval), the animal demonstrated a progressive loss of the anticipatory shift in the 4th to 9th min after reinforcement and developed no such shift prior to the next reinforcement. On return to the 9-min interval, the cat progressively reacquired the anticipatory shift (Figure 54B). This phenomenon has subsequently been demonstrated in three more subjects by Sheafor and Rowland (1973) under even more classical conditions in which the reinforcement was introduced directly into the cat's mouth by an implanted cannula. Two of these subjects graphically demonstrated that the very clear dissociation between the SPS-2 and the mass unit activity (as shown in Figures 53 and 54) depends on a condition Rowland and Sheafor call "quiet expectancy." A frequent pattern was a background of synchronized oscillatory ECoG appearing on the anticipatory slope of the SPS acquired by the cat in temporal conditioning. During this time no sustained change of mass unit activity appeared, the overall integration holding at a constant level. Near the time of reinforcement, however, a spontaneous desynchronization of the oscillogram frequently occurred associated with a conspicuous increment in mass unit activity (Figure 55). The electrooculogram shows movement of the eyes concomitant with the desynchronization and incrementing unit activity. The SPS-2 is seen to be independent of the degree of synchrony of the oscillatory activity (ECoG) and of the integrated massed action potential activity. This suggests an independent SPS-2 genesis that gives information about the animal's processing of the interreinforcement interval different from that found either in the oscillatory ECoG or in the unit activity. Both of these subjects demonstrated responsivity of the units to conditioned auditory stimuli, indicating that the unit activity record was sensitive to environmental stimuli but insensitive to internal conditions related to "quiet expectancy."

Nothing can be stated at this time about the extent to which steady-state phenomena and their shifts, of the kind described here, support, or are supported by, the dynamic pattern theory. Freeman postulates that the steady potential reflects a barrage of inputs biasing the elements receiving them, a process observable by the experimenter with the steady potential but not mediated by the potential itself. If massed unit activity is the criterion of a biasing function of endogenously produced SPS, Rowland sees the dissociations described above as impairing a simple generalization of this kind.

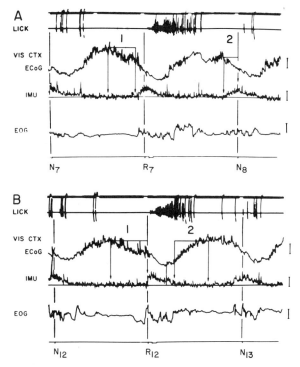

Figure 55. A. A "quiet expectancy" SPS-2 in a cat on a single alternation schedule (N = nonreinforced presentation of 10-sec tone alternating every 2 min with an R trial that is the same 10-sec tone reinforced with food). Signal line pip and verticals through record show onset only of 10-sec tones; 10-sec offset shows duration of food presentation. Numbers refer to trial numbers. Top time line shows seconds and minutes. First bracket indicates quiet expectancy period with constant IMU, synchronized oscillogram, conspicuous SPS-2, and nonmoving eyes as recorded by electrooculogram (EOG). Second bracket shows, by contrast, a period of eye activity and marked increment in IMU activity associated with desynchronized oscillogram and expectancy SPS. VIS CTX = visual cortex. B. Further trials as for A. Typical SPS-2 in a "quiet expectancy" pattern precedes R12 (first bracket) but not, in this case, N13. *During* R12, ECoG desynchronizes and shows SPS-1 associated with a consummatory response and eye activity. After R12, SPS-2 shows a reversal of direction (during restoration to a resting base line) in association with a subsiding but relatively flat IMU. Note that IMU increments are clearly associated with EOG activity, licking, and desynchronization of oscillogram but not with SPS-2. [Rowland]

Interpretation of Two Types of Steady Potential Shift

The appearance of two distinct types of SPS from macroelectrode studies in the awake, behaving animal has not yet been associated with findings from studies at the individual generator level, but the latter investigations, under other conditions, are being advanced by several participants (Grossman, Pollen, and Somjen) at the Work Session.

The marked dissociation between the very responsive SPS generators and the adynamic action potential generators during quiet expectancy, enduring up to 1 to 2 min or more, comes as a surprise. It suggests at least two interpretations, one conventional and the other unconventional but intriguing. Conventionally (based on field response always being the relatively passive consequence of neuronal response), the marked sustained change in steady potential when mass unit activity is unchanged would be seen as the result of the activity of a subset of action potential generators too small or too widely distributed in time to be detected in the mass record. Or, if it is large enough for detection, it is offset by a reciprocal diminution of other action potential generators, leading to no net change in the size of the action potential population sampled by the electrode.

Against this interpretation is the marked association of massed action potential generators with field generators both under conditions of excitation (evoked response, lambda waves, and desynchronization field responses correlating with integrated multiple unit activity (IMU) increments) and inhibition (synchrony and poststimulus "ringing" correlating with IMU decrements). The IMU system developed in these studies is highly sensitive to conditions generating these classical field changes (all of them having noniterated durations under 0.5 sec). Thus, it appears unlikely that the nondetection of IMU change in association with profound sustained field changes having a clearly separated time course (up to minutes) is due to insensitivity of the detecting system.

The unconventionality of the second interpretation lies in its implication that the SPS-2 generators are not only truly dissociated from the massed action potential generators, but can precede action potential patterns by minutes in the state called "quiet expectancy." This has profound implications when one considers that the expectant animal must be relying on a "retrieval" of both immediate and more remote past experience in order to guide the temporal orientation for expectant or anticipatory response. The second interpretation implies that this retrieval process may, under appropriate conditions, occur independently of action potential mediation.

A true understanding of it, of course, must ultimately rely on the identification of the SPS-2 generators. Two leading possibilities are presently entertained: the dendrites of neurons and glial cells. However, other possibilities exist, e.g., another cell population altogether, such as one analogous to Freeman's granule cells in the olfactory system. It appears less likely that the dissociation between SPS-2 and IMU in quiet expectancy is occurring between the dendritic and axonal parts of the neuron than between neurons and glia or some other cell population. Further, neurophysiological studies of Castellucci and Goldring (1970) suggested dendritic SP cannot summate events iterated less frequently than 5/sec.

Against the possibility of glial origin is the long-held view that glia are relatively passively depolarized by neuronal mechanisms and that they metabolically support cells and are not involved in information processing. No electrophysiologic evidence has yet been presented that they are active prior to neuronal response and are a factor in neuronal processing of information. Readily accepted is the likelihood that glia respond to neuronal action through the mediation of extracellular potassium, but what would be the mediating mechanism in the other direction, i.e., from glia to neurons? Although glial hyperpolarization, a presumably active glial mechanism, has been reported (Ransom and Goldring, 1973), it would not guarantee an adequate basis for the mechanism postulated here. It is conceivable that since glia occupy a significant niche, both anatomically and functionally, between capillaries and neurons, they can assert their effects by anticipating the metabolic exchange demands of neurons, and, in order to do this, become an essential repository of information arising from past experience. The acquired change in the SPS-2 generating mechanism, shown with expectancy, is not a static state change like the response of skin with the development of callus that arises with the experience of friction and superficially appears to anticipate the next frictional experience. Rather, the change represents an active response of the generators demonstrating dynamic rather than static anticipation of a forthcoming system change related to environmental stimuli.

Spinal Cord Studies: G. G. Somjen

Somjen (1969, 1970) finds 5-mV extracellular negative shifts in what he calls *sustained* potential* of the spinal cord gray. Induced by electrical stimulus trains to the dorsal root, these shifts are in the negative direction whether neurons are excited or inhibited. Intracellular positive shifts, which always mirror the extracellular negative ones

---

*Also expressed by the abbreviation SPS.

122

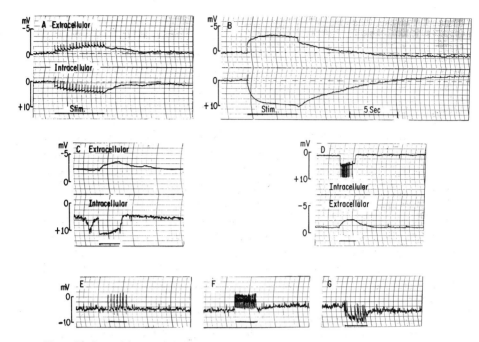

Figure 56. Potentials recorded simultaneously inside and outside cells in the gray matter of the spinal cord, using parallel twin micropipettes whose tips lay about 40 μm apart. A and B. Records from an "unresponsive" (i.e., probably glial) cell. Stimulation of the popliteal nerves: 3/sec in A and 300/sec in B. C to G. Similar records taken from neurons (hyperpolarization in G due to inhibitory input). Note that the sustained shifts of potential recorded inside and outside glial cells are, approximately, mirror images of one another, whereas no such concordance can be detected in recordings made in and outside neurons. [Somjen, 1970]

(Figure 56), are recorded from cells that do not produce action potentials. The ratio of intra- to extracellular SPS amplitude is invariant to thiopental anesthesia and recording site, and maximum amplitudes occur at a constant locus in the spinal cord (see Figures 57 to 61). Also, the SPS's are not correlated with membrane potential changes of neurons. In Somjen's view, these observations support the probable glial origin of SPS in the spinal cord.

Despite the larger magnitude of spinal cord SPS's compared to those observed in the cortex, the cord is resistant to spreading depression and seizures. According to Somjen (1973), this may be pointing towards definition of the essential properties and structure necessary for the development of what we refer to as pathological dynamic patterns (see discussions of Ferguson and Van Harreveld below).

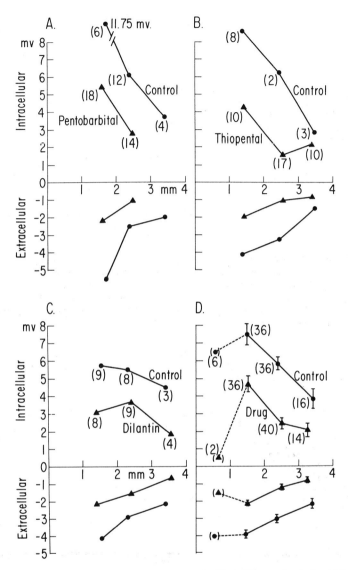

Figure 57. Averaged depolarization evoked by standardized afferent stimulation of "unresponsive" cells found at varying depths in the spinal cord, and the corresponding SPS recorded in their neighborhood, before and after the administration of depressant drugs. A. Results pooled from 4 experiments, before and after 30 to 60 mg/kg of pentobarbital. B. From 6 experiments, 25 to 50 mg/kg of thiopental. C. From 4 experiments, 20 to 40 mg/kg of diphenylhydantoin (Dilantin). D. From all experiments (A to C) combined. Vertical bars show standard errors of means. Symbols indicate mean value from cells found within 1-mm micrometer readings; abscissal position of symbols shows mean depth of cells. Numbers in parentheses indicate number of cells in each group. [Strittmatter and Somjen, 1973]

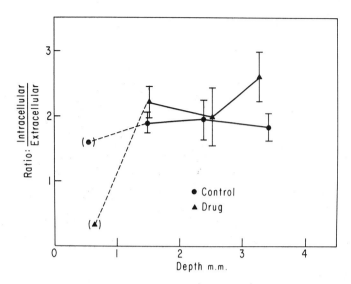

Figure 58. Ratio of depolarizing shift of membrane potential of "unresponsive" cells and corresponding extracellular SPS, before and after administation of depressant drugs. Derived from same measurements as given in Figure 57, D. Vertical bars show standard errors of means. Symbols shown in parentheses for "drugged" cells found above a 1-mm depth represent two measurements only and are not considered reliable. Differences between control and "drugged" values are statistically not significant ($P > 0.1$). [Strittmatter and Somjen, 1973]

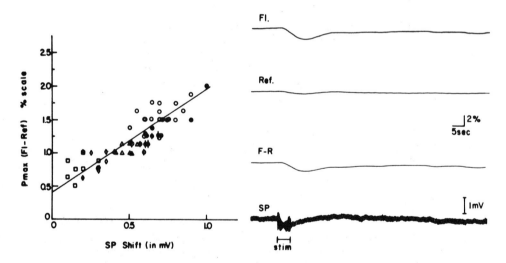

Figure 59. A. Metabolic activity and sustained potential shift of the cerebral cortex. Method of Jöbsis and co-workers (1971) was used to estimate NADH levels in the intact cortex. Corrected fluorescence, at its point of maximal deflection (P_{max}), measured at 450 nm (F-R on the tracings) was taken to be a measure of intramitochondrial NADH and, hence, of oxidative metabolic activity. Graph in the upper left part of the figure shows oxidative activity plotted against SPS evoked by repetitive stimulation of the cortical surface. Note the linear correlation. Tracings in the right part of the figure show sample recordings for the graph at the left. [Rosenthal and Somjen, 1973]

124

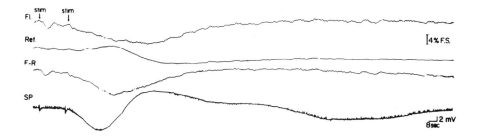

Figure 59. B. Recordings taken during spreading depression evoked by direct stimulation of the cortical surface (at the arrows marked "stim"). Note that there is apparently no shortage of oxidizable substrate at the moment when spreading depression erupts. Note also an unusually intensive metabolic response accompanying the depressive process. Fl. = fluorescence, Ref. = reflectance, F.S. = fluorescence signal. [Rosenthal and Somjen, 1973]

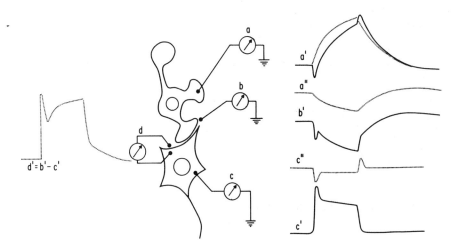

Figure 60. Proposed mechanism of sustained potential shifts evoked by afferent stimulation in the spinal gray matter. a, b, c, and d indicate modes of recording from glia (a), from neurons (c and d), and from extracellular space (b). Solid lines of a', b', and c' are "idealized" versions of potential shifts frequently recorded near the base of the dorsal horn and intermediate gray matter (positivity upwards). Broken line of a' shows suggested "pure" glial depolarization, presumably caused by a raised extracellular K^+ level. a" indicates the contribution of glia to extracellular potential. c" shows suggested contribution of the sustained synaptic current (EPSP) of neurons to extracellular potential. The deviation of the solid line from the broken line in a' arises, presumably, by the action of extracellular current generated by neurons upon the membrane potential of glia. b' is composite of a" and c" and corresponds to an actually registered typical SPS. d' shows a transmembrane potential of a neuron with depolarization plotted upwards. [Somjen, 1970]

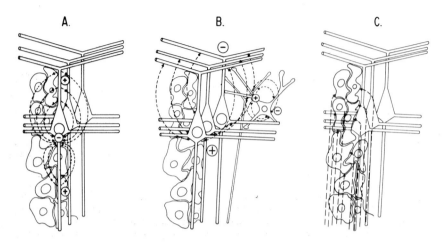

A.   B.   C.

Figure 61. Schema of extracellular currents in central nervous tissue. A. When a nerve impulse is born at the axon hillock, it draws extracellular current from the cell soma, dendrites, and the inactive portion of the axon. There is an intense but localized sink and weak, widely dispersed sources of current. B. If many neurons are similarly aligned and are generating synaptic currents, they can create extracellular fields which are detectable over a wide area. Transmembrane synaptic potentials are of smaller amplitude than action potentials, but synaptic potentials last longer and are distributed over wider parts of the cells' surfaces than are spike potentials; hence, the former are relatively more effective generators of extracellular current than the latter. Neurons that do not conform to the spatial "register," such as the single cells shown in the background of the diagram in B, and neurons that are activated "out of turn" can distort extracellular synaptic current fields. C. The contribution of glial cells to extracellular current. Glial cells in the upper part of the figure that lie near active neurons, and are therefore exposed to a concentration of K^+ higher than that in the "resting" state, are depolarized and draw current from glia lying in an inactive region. The current must return through an intracellular path (not shown in diagram) either by way of intercellular electrotonic junctions or through long, filamentous processes of glial cells. [Somjen, 1973]

Extracellular Potassium and Steady Potential:
E. Eidelberg

The extent to which the glial cell is to be considered a relatively active or passive generator of steady or sustained potential is unresolved, and contrasting arguments were presented at the Work Session. Pollen commented that glia may act passively to extracellular K^+ concentrations varying with neuronal activity. This view was affirmed by Eidelberg, who thinks that the extracellular K^+ concentration is the most parsimoniously conceived generator of steady potentials (SP). This is based on the discrepancy between the neuronal membrane potentials recorded intracellularly in the cortex and the predicted (20 to 30 mV higher) value for them, based on a 20-fold intracellular/

extracellular concentration ratio for potassium (K_i/K_o). According to Eidelberg's hypothesis, this difference is accounted for most simply by an electrogenic pump for K^+ similar to the "driving potential" described by Ussing and his collaborators in frog skin preparations (Ussing and Zerahn, 1951; Bricker et al., 1963). This hypothesis, emphasizing the role of extracellular K^+, is not viewed by him as contradicting the possible role of glia as passively responding to neuronally generated K^+_o changes. Neurons are assumed to be the primary generators of the changes because SP changes are produced by synaptically mediated inputs to the cortex (Arduini, 1958; Gumnit, 1960; see also Rowland above). The question then arises: Why is the SP recorded by electrodes that are not selective for K^+ attributed only to K_o levels? Vyškoćil and his colleagues (1972) have recently shown that, in fact, SP changes are closely paralleled by extracellular K^+ changes measured directly by selective electrodes. This occurred in terms of very large shifts induced by anoxia and spreading depression. Secondly, in Eidelberg's (1962) experiments, changes in concentration of other ions did not significantly affect SP levels, while the SP was a linear function of the logarithm of the K^+ concentration, thus establishing that the species of ion and not just its charge is the significant factor.

However, it is the second part of Eidelberg's hypothesis that is more relevant to the theme of the meeting. Immature cortex (Eidelberg et al., 1965; Deza and Eidelberg, 1967) and adult cortex pretreated with solutions of high Ca^{2+} concentration (Bureš and Burešová, 1956; Eidelberg, 1962) respond to K^+ increases in the manner described above. Adult "normal" cortex does so up to a "threshold" SP level, beyond which a regenerative process, all-or-nothing in character, develops much beyond the subthreshold event. Further, it moves away from the site of initiation and may recur cyclically (the classical spreading depression, SD, of Leão). It has been proposed by Grafstein (1956) that the movement of the SD wave reflects a chain of neuronal excitation processes linked by K^+ release. In Eidelberg's view SD represents a good model of a cooperative process in neural masses. While this situation is definitely pathological, direct-coupled recording from the cortex shows that in "normal" conditions SP changes of much smaller amplitude not only occur but appear to be linked to higher neural processes (Gumnit, 1960; also Rowland above). Eidelberg concludes that SP changes perhaps related to K^+ concentration waves, rather than purely diffusional events (Othmer and Scriven, 1971), may serve functionally to regulate and modify neuronal excitability levels in relatively large populations, in addition to classical synaptic routes.

Cortical Glial Studies: R. G. Grossman

At the Work Session, Grossman reviewed the following: (1) evidence for astrocytic (glial) participation in carbon dioxide, chloride, potassium, and water exchange, (2) the possibility of glia being one of several removal paths for neuronally created increments in extracellular potassium, (3) the possible responsiveness of glia to a neurotransmitter (norepinephrine), and (4) the possible participation of glia in controlling vascular channels and oscillations of oxygen levels (see Rowland above and Table 3). He cited the carbonic anhydrase content of glia and its role in the development of brain swelling (water influx) due to KCl uptake (Bourke et al., 1970). All these observations point towards a specialization of glial functions around their sensitivity to extracellular potassium. This emphasis contrasts with the passive role of glia with respect to potassium as implied by Eidelberg's hypothesis (see above).

In cortex "silent cells," from which the neuronal population has been reduced by cold-induced lesions, Grossman and Rosman (1971) observed that direct cortical electrical stimulation can induce initial depolarizing shifts, followed by up to 10-mV hyperpolarizing shifts enduring up to 1 min after stimulation. Hyperpolarization of the presumed glial cell is not found in cold-blooded animals, but it is seen in silent cells in the cat following natural spindle-burst activity, as well as after direct cortical stimulation. Grossman stated that it is premature to regard the hyperpolarization as representing active ion pumping by glia, but it might be related to uptake of a negative ion, such as Cl^-, after being exposed to an excess of positive ion (Figures 62-65).

A major difficulty in understanding glial dynamics is the uncertainty concerning the electrical characteristics of the glial membrane and, therefore, of the way currents flow in and around it. Grossman finds that the time constant of the membrane of "silent cells" in the cat cortex, which are presumed to be glia, probably astrocytes, is little more than that of the pipette with which he measures it, namely, 180 to 400 μsec, and the input resistance of the cells is 1.5 to 8 MΩ. Resistance is lowest for the cells with the highest membrane potentials.

The specific resistance of the membrane of the presumed glia from which the recordings were made cannot be calculated directly because of the uncertainty of the surface area of the cells recorded from. However, as pointed out by Trachtenberg and Pollen (1970), the

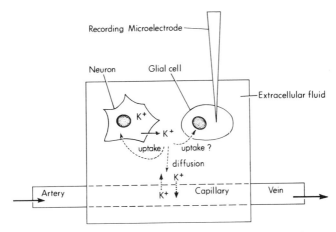

Figure 62. Model of the mechanism of depolarization of a glial cell by K⁺ liberated from neurons and possible pathways of K⁺ uptake. [Grossman, 1972b]

small time constant of these cells suggests that their membranes have a low specific resistance. Grossman cites further that input resistivity could be low not only because of the intrinsic properties of the membrane, but also because of low-resistance gap junctions between glial cells. Also, according to Pollen, different values may also be related to variations in the species and types of glial cell used, i.e., whether the glia are of the fibrous or protoplasmic type. There appears, however, to be general agreement that the value of the membrane time constant for neocortical neuroglial cells is some 20-fold less than that for the pyramidal cells in cat neocortex (Trachtenberg and Pollen, 1970).

Pollen contended that glial cells are unlikely generators of extracellular potentials, because their membrane resistance is very low. In responding to this contention, Somjen pointed out that a low-membrane resistance is not an impediment to the generation of extracellular current, and, hence, of extracellular potential gradients. He cited the development of a computer-simulated model of a network of electrotonically connected glia cells in which simulated extracellular SPS's grow in amplitude, but become more locally concentrated with steeper gradients between excited and resting regions when, other variables remaining constant, the membrane resistance is lowered (Joyner and Somjen, 1972; see the Appendix to Somjen, 1973). In other words, membrane resistance principally affects the "space constant" of SPS. The main indispensable condition for glia to generate extracellular current is electrotonic continuity between depolarized and "resting" areas; small cells, insulated one from the other, cannot create

130

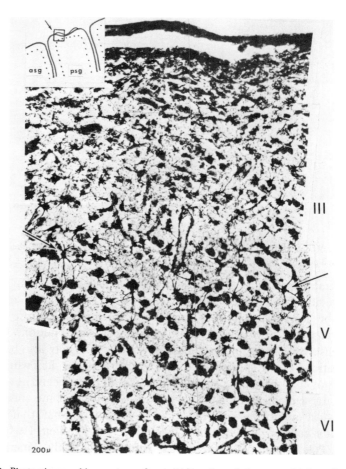

Figure 63. Photomicrographic montage of a sagittal section of the cortex 30 days after cold injury showing hypertrophied astrocytes. Intracellular recordings were obtained from "silent cells" presumed to be glia in this type of gliotic cortex. The area of the posterior sigmoid gyrus (psg) shown is indicated in the drawing of the sagittal section of the sigmoid gyri. The montage shows a transitional zone of damage lying between the margin of the lesion on the left and the center of the lesion at the atrophic crest of the psg, which lies to the right of the montage. The approximate depth of cell layers III, V, and VI is indicated. Note that severe damage to the upper cortical layers increases in depth going from the periphery towards the center of the lesion. Two very large reactive astrocytes lying at the lower margin of severely damaged cortex are marked by arrows. Tsujiyama's (1963) method for staining macroglia. asg = anterior sigmoid gyrus. [Grossman and Rosman, 1971]

SPS. Intracellular electrotonic continuity can be provided either by long cellular processes (as shown by Ramón y Cajal, 1955) or by intercellular electrical junctions (Kuffler et al., 1966).

Computer simulation also demonstrated that, when extra-cellular current is drawn from glial cells, the change of potential

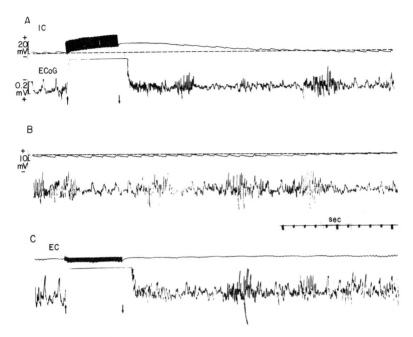

Figure 64. Depolarizing and late, slow, hyperpolarizing potentials of an inexcitable cell in gliotic cortex. Resting membrane potential (86 mV) penetrated at a depth of 150 μm, 20 days after cold injury. A and B. Continuous oscillograph recording. Upper line, intracellular potentials (IC); lower line, electrocorticogram (ECoG). Stimulation of the cortex at 40/sec during the interval marked by the arrows. C. Extracellular potentials recorded with the micropipette withdrawn from the cell (EC). [Grossman and Rosman, 1971]

measured across the cell membrane is reduced, because "resting" cells then act as an electrical shunt for depolarizing tissue elements. Under these circumstances, unlike those of tissue in an isolated organ bath, glial membrane potential can no longer accurately reflect changes of extracellular potassium concentration. In sum, glia can either be a precise "potassium electrode" or a generator of extracellular SPS, but not both at once.

Grossman also noted the observation of Ramón y Cajal (1955) that astrocytes of the external glial limiting membrane have vertically oriented fibers extending a considerable distance with respect to the cortical surface. According to Grossman, these fibers could produce the large, surface-recorded extracellular currents observed. The glia could differentially depolarize at the lower levels of cortex where neuronal activity is intense and convey, via the vertical fibers, the currents

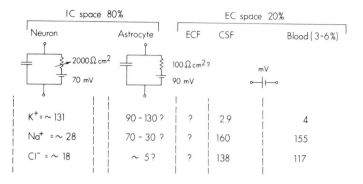

Figure 65. Intracellular and extracellular compartments of brain tissue. An equivalent circuit for neurons and a probable equivalent circuit for astrocytes are shown. Probable ionic concentrations are shown in milliequivalents per liter. IC = intracellular; EC = extracellular; ECF = extracellular fluid; CSF = cerebrospinal fluid. Based on data obtained from body fluids and motor cortex of the cat. [Grossman, 1972a]

flowing towards the cortical surface. It is thus possible that a K^+ ion path leading to the cortical surface would lead to K^+ movement into the CSF.

Influence of Exogenous Low-Level Currents

The extent to which a weak steady current applied to the brain simulates the natural phenomenon of a steady potential shift remains controversial. In the context of the central importance of a dissipation of free energy in the emergence and maintenance of dynamic patterns, one might expect such currents to modify the dissipative flows in hypothetical neural dynamic patterns. No direct evidence, however, exists that this is the modus operandi of SPS. Weak polarizations have been shown, however, to have "learning-like" neural effects that outlast, by up to 40 min, the period of polarization and then decay.

Electrophysiological Effects of Direct Currents: F. Morrell

At the most elementary level it is easy to demonstrate that anodal polarization increases the firing rate of many cells (Figure 66) and that this increase relates directly to current density. Such observations are in accord with eighteen published reports by various investigators from 1952 to 1967. Creutzfeldt and his co-workers (1962) felt that naturally occurring SP gradients were too small by a

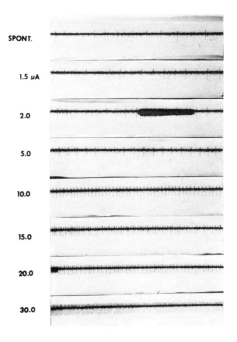

SPONT.

1.5 µA

2.0

5.0

10.0

15.0

20.0

30.0

Figure 66. Effect of various levels of anodal polarization of the crayfish abdominal ganglion on the firing rate of a spontaneously active crayfish axon. Currents applied are directly translatable to current density in terms of $\mu A/mm^2$. [K.L. Chow and A.L. Leiman, unpublished studies]

factor of 10 to 20 to be seriously considered as effectors of neuronal activity. They did not use intracellular recordings or examine synaptic potentials. Purpura and McMurtry (1965) have also noted that low-level polarization has little effect on action potential genesis in the pyramidal cell. At the same time, Purpura emphasized significant alteration of synaptic activity, and of firing rate as well, in nonpyramidal neurons nearer to the cortical surface (and therefore to the polarizing electrode). It seems somewhat arbitrary to assume that initiation of all-or-none action potentials in large pyramidal neurons should be the sole criterion of effectiveness. The argument seems even less cogent when one considers that the most interesting effects of polarizing currents (see below) are attributable to alteration in synaptic events of exactly the sort which Purpura and McMurtry (1965) have shown to be directly influenced by low-level dc currents. Furthermore, since it is now generally established that EEG rhythms are themselves consequences of synaptic activity, we may accept the extensive investigations of polarization effects on EEG and evoked potentials as evidence for an impact of low-level dc gradients on synaptic processes.

Higher Order Effects

Other observations on cellular activity in cortical fields subject to low-level dc polarization have persistent, long-lasting features that suggest an effect on other than all-or-none electrogenic tissue. Morrell presented several kinds of patterns of which the following are representative. Figure 67 illustrates poststimulus time (PST) histograms from a visual cortical cell stroboscopically stimulated at a frequency of 10 Hz. The first summation of 20 trials did not reveal acquisition of the stimulus rhythm, but, clearly, by the third summation (Trials 41-60), the cellular firing pattern exhibited the expected entrainment. At that point the stimulus frequency was dropped to 1/sec and was so maintained for the duration of observation of this cell. It took virtually 60 trials (Trials 61-120) before the 10/sec pattern was obliterated. The existence of the steady potential gradient appears to be crucial to (1) the striking fidelity of initial entrainment (Trials 1-60) and (2) the

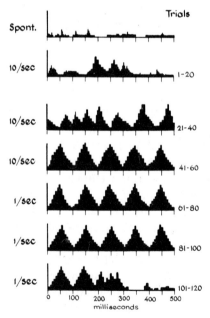

Figure 67. PST histograms of the firing pattern of an assimilation cell recorded at a depth of 0.9 mm in the right anterior marginal gyrus of an unanesthetized, paralyzed cat. Surface anodal polarization was 10 μA/mm^2 and was applied throughout the experiment. Stroboscopic stimulus frequency labeled on the left; trial numbers on the right. Trace labeled "spont." = 20 sweeps triggered in the same way but without a light flash. Bar at time zero = 20 counts; bin width = 5 msec. [Morrell]

persistence of that pattern despite the change in stimulus frequency (Trials 61-100).

Morrell attributes the above type of response to what he calls an assimilation cell. He finds another type, referred to as a doublet cell, that, on low-level polarization, gives a briefly persisting doublet response after double-flash stimulation has been terminated and that resumes with a doublet response when single flashes are started. These polarized cells demonstrate the peculiar "inertia" of the response process noted in anodally polarized neuronal populations. The term "inertia" is used to describe a response pattern that, once established (for instance, a doublet response to double-flash stimulation), tends to persist even when the stimulus is changed to a single flash. Eventually, the cell "catches on" and switches to a single spike configuration. The term "inertia" is used descriptively only and does not imply any knowledge of the basic neural mechanisms involved. It might be pointed out that the word "hysteresis" would be equally applicable and perhaps more appropriate (though less biological) to these discussions.

Another measure of the change of state of a system is the duration of stimulation necessary to trigger a "photic driving" response.* For example, a cell was found that responded well to flash frequencies of 4/sec and 7/sec (Figure 68). Both frequencies were tested for their capacity to induce photic driving prior to application of the anodal current (Figure 68, left). During polarization only the 7/sec stimulus frequency was used. Systematic diminution of the time required to induce driving was noted (curve in center of Figure 68). The dc polarization was then terminated and the two original frequencies were compared with respect to effectiveness in eliciting "driving" responses. The right-hand portion of Figure 68 tells the tale; the cell remained tuned, i.e., selectively sensitive to the frequency administered during anodal polarization. Response to the 4/sec flash was essentially the same as that during the prepolarization period. Thus, in some manner, the imposed electrical field conferred upon the affected cells the capacity of retaining for some time a representation of the stimulus configuration paired with polarization—a finding reminiscent of the observation that a motor cortical cell could be activated selectively by an acoustical signal that had been presented during anodal polarization but was unaffected by an equally loud but novel sound (Morrell, 1961a).

---

*Driving is defined as continuously following the stimulus frequency for 10 sec.

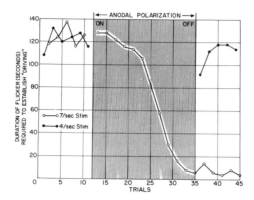

Figure 68. Differentiation of response frequency by low-level anodal polarization. This cell responded to both 4/sec and 7/sec flashes before exposure to polarizing current. Equally long conditioning periods (duration of flashing before "driving" appears) were needed for the two stimuli. The 7/sec stimulus was then repeatedly presented during imposition of a steady potential gradient and the curve exhibited progressive diminution. Following cessation of polarization, it was possible to test both stimulus frequencies, i.e., the 7/sec which had combined with polarization and the 4/sec which had not. The duration of the 7/sec stimulation needed to induce driving continued to be low, whereas the duration of the 4/sec stimulation remained high and essentially at control levels. [Morrell]

Gross electrical rhythms yielded similar sensitivity to low-level polarization. A study of this kind involves pairing of stroboscopic flicker (unconditional stimulus (UCS)) with a steady tone (conditional stimulus (CS)) in the manner shown in Figure 69. The Stage I conditional electrocortical response, which occurs only in the interval between the onset of the tone and the onset of the flicker, consisted of generalized desynchronization in all cortical regions. In Stage II the acoustical signal gave rise during the tone-light interval to a repetitive series of waves in the visual cortex at, or close to, the frequency of the intermittent light. The Stage II response lasted for only 10 to 20 trials, after which it gave way to the Stage III response in which the conditional acoustical signal provoked a localized desynchronization in visual cortical derivations. Although the Stage III response was the most stable, in a strict Pavlovian sense the Stage II response was the one most characteristic of conditioning. Only during Stage II did the conditional electrocortical response replicate the unconditional response. Why doesn't it persist?

Some years ago Konorski suggested that the feature that biologically significant reinforcers might possibly have in common was the establishment of an enduring steady potential gradient. It seemed logical, therefore, to apply surface anodal polarization at levels

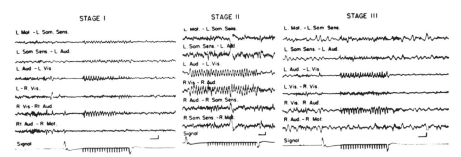

Figure 69. Examples of EEG tracings from surface cortical electrodes for each of three stages of electrocortical conditioning. Derivations are from implanted electrodes at the sites indicated in an unanesthetized animal. First upward deflection on the signal channel indicates the onset of a 500 CPS tone. A photocell records the stroboscopic flashes superimposed upon the signal line. The final downward deflection indicates cessation of the tone and light. Calibration = 50 μV and 1 sec. Stages I, II, and III are explained in the text. [Morrell, 1966]

previously shown to have effects both on single units (Morrell, 1961a) and behavior (Rusinov, 1953; Morrell and Naitoh, 1962).

The results obtained from two different cats are illustrated in Figure 70. A computer recorded half-period counts of a 6/sec (UCS) rhythm during the CS interval. Thus, the occurrence of Stage II conditional electrocortical response without polarization (Day 1) did not persist. Application of anodal current resulted in an earlier appearance of the conditional electrocortical response (approximately Trial 44) that persisted for about 100 trials. Results on the second day were even more dramatic, and on Day 3 the Stage II response was present in virtually all trials even in the absence of polarization. The latter observation argues strongly against interpreting the Day 2 finding as an instance of state-dependent learning. Had polarization never been used, the incidence of Stage II response would be at the level indicated by the unshaded (control) portion of the graph. Similar data from a second animal are charted in Figure 70B. These findings verify Konorski's prediction and thus support his hunch.

Morrell observes that electrical fields exist in the central nervous system at levels appreciably higher than those which Terzuolo and Bullock (1956) suggested as adequate to modulate neuronal firing in invertebrate ganglia, i.e., 1 mV/mm. Indeed, the firing of a single anterior horn cell produces a field of 5 to 10 times that level (Fatt, 1957; Nelson and Frank, 1964) and has been demonstrated to modify the excitability of an adjacent cell by as much as 30% (Nelson, 1966). Furthermore, Nelson (1966) has pointed out that the geometry of the spinal cord is much less favorable than that of laminated and radially

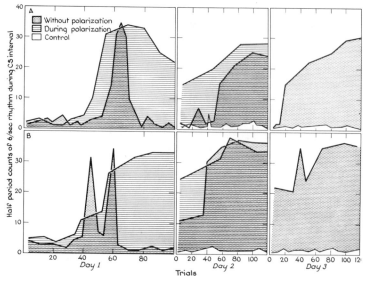

Figure 70. Electrocortical conditioning for 3 days in two separate cats, A (*upper*) and B (*lower*). Incidence of half-period counts of a 6/sec (the UCS) rhythm on each trial. Without polarization the occurrence of a Stage II response (high counts) was limited to a single peak between about Trial 50-70 in cat A and to two peaks each of even briefer duration in cat B. With polarization, on the other hand, the Stage II response began earlier and persisted throughout the day. The next day a Stage II response was established early and strongly even without polarization but earlier and stronger with it. On Day 3 no polarization was used, but the Stage II response was present nearly all of the time. If there had been no polarization at all, the response level expected is that shown in the white (control) section at the bottom. [Morrell]

oriented structures like hippocampus or neocortex both for generation of potential fields and for their appreciation by adjacent cells. Effects of comparable magnitude have been demonstrated in medullated nerve (Arvanitaki, 1942; Katz and Schmitt, 1942; Granit and Skoglund, 1945). (For pharmacological studies on spinal cord and cortex having similar implications, see Bernhard, 1958.)

The SP shifts recorded naturally may be epiphenomena rather than causally related to behavior. Similarities between naturally occurring gradients and artificial polarizing currents may be more apparent than real especially in the details of field structure and organization. Changes induced by artificial polarization, therefore, may be unrelated in mechanism to those which normally mediate processes like consolidation. On the other hand, if SP fields do play a role in neural integrative activity, it would seem most likely that their action is mediated through effects on synaptic function. For that reason it seems pertinent to review and compare some of the limited data available

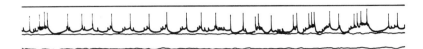

Figure 71. Spontaneous activity of a visual neuron (unidentified except that it responded to visual stimulation within a precisely defined receptive field) encountered at 0.9 mm beneath the pial surface in area 18. Surface anodal current $(10\ \mu A/mm^2)$ applied through a Ag-AgCl electrode having a surface area of 5 mm². Current had been on for about 25 min before impalement of this cell. Note the showers of fast prepotentials. The top channel had been displaced from the third channel by 50 mV and serves as a voltage calibration. [Morrell]

from intracellular studies that point to a particular kind and direction of change in synaptic function which seems especially appropriate if, in real life, SP fields have something to do with the consolidation of experience.

Observations made independently in Morrell's laboratory and in that of Purpura are so concordant that it seems difficult to believe that they arise by chance. Thus, Purpura and McMurtry (1965) demonstrate an enduring enhancement of excitatory postsynaptic potentials in a nonpyramidal tract cell of low-level surface anodal current, which Morrell believes indicates an alteration in synaptic efficacy. The effect persisted for 20 sec after cessation of cortical polarization.

Other signs of exalted excitability were also reported by Purpura and McMurtry (1965), such as the occurrence of fast prepotentials in a nonpyramidal tract cell. These events have been interpreted as dendritic spikes by Spencer and Kandel (1961b).

It is interesting to compare these findings with the fast prepotentials shown in the intracellular record (Figure 71) of a visual neuron in an anodally polarized field studied in Morrell's laboratory. Occurrence of fast prepotentials is sufficiently unusual in normal adult cortical (nonhippocampal) neurons to make the concordance seem unlikely to be attributable to chance and more likely to relate to the common experimental variable of cortical polarization.

Mechanisms Involved in the Actions of Weak Polarizing Currents

While these preliminary observations have not yet provided major insights into the mechanism, it seems fair to state that the main impact of a surface-to-depth, radially oriented potential field is on synaptic processes (perhaps presynaptic terminals as well as post-synaptic membrane) in dendritic arborizations at a considerable distance from sites of action potential genesis in deep-lying cell somata. Since it has been shown that surface-positive polarization is excitatory and is believed to facilitate learning, it seems especially appropriate that this *direction* of change in synaptic function induced by surface anodal current is an *augmentation of transmission efficacy,* an augmentation that is slow and gradual in onset and prolonged in duration of polarization by seconds to several minutes. Although none of these observations taken individually can be regarded as providing hard evidence, taken together, they are sufficiently suggestive as to warrant much more detailed investigation than they have so far received.

Morrell postulated several possible mechanisms for the effects of weak anodal polarization: (1) membrane reactions on the dendritic tree, (2) changes in transmitter release by action of the current on fine terminals, (3) migration of divalent cations in a weak polarizing field causing local concentrations and facilitating synthesis or release of transmitters (calcium is known to effect transmitter release), and (4) effects on neuronal membrane having known high electrical resistance when that neuronal membrane resistance is momentarily low at the time of action potential genesis. It is also possible that an effect arises on glial membranes. Katchalsky commented that conformational changes in possibly acidic protein could be "frozen in" by a weak polarizing current and endure for long periods.

Are Weak Oscillating Fields Detected By the Brain? W. R. Adey

Responses of monkeys and cats to weak oscillatory electric fields in air were described in experiments by Adey and his colleagues and support the possibility of direct interaction of these fields with brain tissue (Gavalas et al., 1970). In monkeys exposed to a 7 Hz electric field at an intensity of 100 mV/cm (Figure 72), there was a significant shortening of subjective estimates of the passage of time (Figure 73). There were concomitant changes in EEG activity at 7 Hz in hippocampal structures, which characteristically show theta rhythms around this frequency. The EEG changes appeared gradually in the course of field exposure (Gavalas et al., 1970). No changes in time estimation were noted with 10 Hz fields; however, Wever (1968) has reported accelerated circadian rhythms in men exposed to 10 Hz fields with a gradient of 25 mV/cm. In cats exposed to 147 MHz fields, amplitude-modulated at frequencies between 3 and 16 Hz (Figure 74) and with the same magnitude of electric field (100 mV/cm), specific sleep states were induced, and internal brain rhythms used as conditional responses were much modified (Bawin et al., 1973).

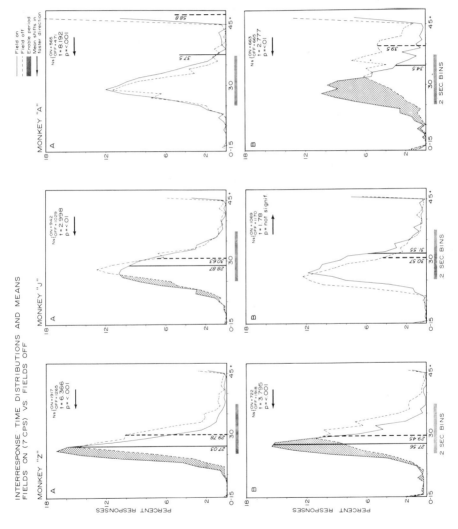

Figure 72. Behavioral data showing shifts in interresponse time under 7 Hz fields. The abscissa shows time between responses in 0.2-sec bins; the ordinate shows percent of total responses at each interval. (Note that only bins 15-45 are plotted; bins 0-144 were used in calculation of means and standard deviations.) [Gavalas et al., 1970]

141

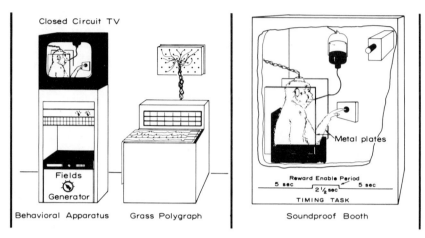

Figure 73. Experimental paradigm used in exposing monkeys to low-level, low-frequency oscillating electric fields. Electrode plates 50 cm² were placed on either side of the monkey's chair, with a plate separation of 40 cm. The electric gradient was between 25 and 100 mV/cm at either 7 or 10 Hz. Behavioral and EEG changes were seen with 7 Hz fields, but not with 10 Hz fields. The monkey was rewarded with apple juice for estimating the passage of 5 sec within a 2.5-sec "enable" period. A similar arrangement of plates was used in the modulated very high frequency studies of Bawin and co-workers (1973). [Gavalas et al., 1970]

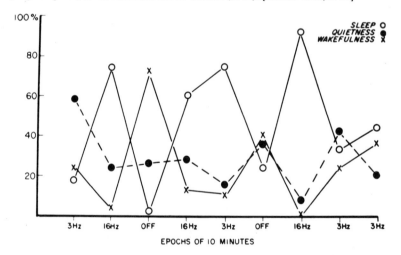

Figure 74. Effects of amplitude-modulated 147 MHz fields on alertness levels in the cat. The very high frequency field had an incident energy of approximately 1 mV/cm² (electric gradient in air, 100 mV/cm). Amplitude modulation level of carrier wave was 90%. Modulation at 3 Hz was characterized by development of EEG slow wave patterns and associated with behavioral deep sleep. Modulation at 16 Hz was accompanied by development of rapid eye movement (REM) sleep. Unmodulated fields were without effects on EEG or behavior. Modulated fields greatly increased time-to-extinction of conditional EEG responses, where the evoked EEG response and the modulation frequencies were closely related. [Bawin et al., 1973]

Unmodulated, very high-frequency fields were without effect on EEG or behavior. For the low-frequency fields, actual measurement of current flow to ground from a "phantom" monkey head placed in the field was 0.8 nA.

Cooperativity as a Mechanism for Field Effects

Adey proposed that these electrophysiological, biochemical, and behavioral effects of weak electric fields in central nervous tissue may arise in processes that are cooperatively organized on at least two levels. At a molecular level, cationic interactions with polyanionic surface macromolecules may be optimal at "patches" of membrane that exhibit a temporary cooperativity between adjacent fixed charges, as suggested by Schwarz (1970). At a much higher level, interaction between cellular elements in a cortical domain may occur through mutual sensitivity to weak electric fields that are produced in part by these elements of the domain itself.

Evidence Contradicting Neuron Sensitivity to Extracellular Fields

Purpura remarked that he had abandoned weak polarizing approaches because of the following problems: (1) the unknown "leakage" of currents in many directions, (2) the lack of control of currents in relation to the cell under observation, and (3) the absence of any effect on the action potential genesis of the pyramidal cell. He confirmed that weak polarizations profoundly affected dendritic events without affecting action potential firing.

Pollen reviewed the consensus of electrophysiologists on the insensitivity of neurons to extracellular exogenous currents which must be 25- to 40-fold greater than those (1×10^{-9} A) that determine the action potential genesis when delivered inside the cell, regardless of current density considerations. By these criteria, he finds field potentials and associated currents to be implausible communication paths. In his opinion, they are much too weak to account for the information-processing functions of neurons.

Pollen thinks that the dynamic pattern theory can be appropriately applied to subatomic systems (e.g., electron-positron pair formation in the electron vacuum), but, once atomic and molecular structures are established from subatomic entities, the theory would have, at best, utility only of the second or third order and be of relatively little value. When similarly applied to the nervous system, the dynamic pattern concept, although potentially important in morphogenesis, can be only of secondary or tertiary importance because structural connectivity, once established, would be the primary determinant in an information-processing system that is widely distributed and resistant to nonlinearities and distortions.

These important criticisms underscore the necessity for clarifying the view that the dynamic pattern concept is not concerned with overthrowing connectionism or establishing that fields are a significant driving force in the nervous system. The Bénard and Belousov-Zhabotinsky demonstrations indicate that stable organizations can arise dynamically out of relative homogeneity at levels of chemical organization (atoms and molecules) well above the subatomic levels to which Pollen would limit the concept. The Wilson and Cowan (1972) model demonstrates at least the theoretical applicability of the concept to a system that is, by definition, connectionist. The concept may possibly be applicable to the nervous system's distributivity and resistance to nonlinearities as stressed by Pollen, and it may even complement our understanding of these properties in its emphasis on the mechanism by which stable (i.e., resistant to perturbation) regions of operation are achieved and maintained.

The question arose whether electrical recording is insensitive to an order of magnitude of chemical interactions well below the changes observed electrophysiologically. Adey affirms this on the basis of cyclic AMP amplification effects, membrane sensitivity to molecular concentrations being as low as 10^{-14}M.* Weak polarizations, such as those used by Morrell, could be exerting effects below the electrically demonstrable range. Bennett commented that effects too small to be seen electrically in a single cell may be noted by observing a population of cells with an implied summation effect. The question thus raised is whether summation is the only collective property to be examined since it is not adequate if the elemental processes to be combined are nonlinear. Purpura wondered how the problems can be advanced when, for example, there are several different kinds of spines seen on cerebellar cells and the same fields hitting them could produce very different effects.

---

*Although neurotransmitter interactions usually require neurotransmitter concentrations on the order of 10^{-5}M, membrane responses to hormones and pheromones are much more sensitive, ranging from 10^{-11}M for insulin (Cuatrecasas, 1971) to 10^{-13}M for ACTH (Sayers and Beall, 1973), and to 2×10^{-17}M for bombykol pheromone (Kaissling, 1971).

Pathologic Dynamic Patterns

Acetylcholine-Induced Seizure Activity: J. H. Ferguson

In addition to the potential usefulness of the dynamic pattern concept in physiological processes are its possibilities for furthering our understanding of pathologic mechanisms such as epilepsy. Studies of the continuously recurring paroxysmal pattern of the deep cortical negative shift with secondary oscillations that emerges in the cortex after the topical placement of acetylcholine (ACh) with neostigmine have been carried out by Ferguson (1972a,b; Ferguson and Jasper, 1971; Ferguson and Cornblath, 1974)(see Figure 75A). The pattern

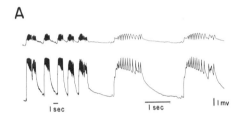

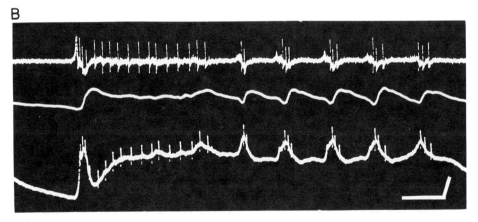

Figure 75. A. Epileptiform activity following application of ACh. *Top,* surface macroelectrode and *bottom,* microelectrode recording field in layer V of suprasylvian cortex. Slow paper speed on the left; 1-mV calibration for both traces; negative is up. Note clock-like, repetitive burst paroxysms, large negative dc shift in depths, and interparoxysmal intervals without oscillations. B. Unit recording, depth 1570 μm, during one ACh paroxysm. *Upper,* unit record, rc-coupled amplifier; *middle,* surface record; *lower,* microelectrode at micrometer depth of 1570 μm, dc-coupled. Note unit silence at left corresponding to interparoxysmal interval, and unit synchrony at onset of a negative dc shift and with depth-negative portions of each oscillation. [Ferguson]

appears in normal cortex and can still be demonstrated in either an acutely or chronically undercut cortex preparation. The acutely undercut cortex preparation shows, by a striking absence of action potential activity, an unexpected dissociation between field and action potentials. In the intact or chronically undercut cortex, fields, unit activity, and unit silence correlate regularly irrespective of depth of units (Figure 75B). This ubiquitous on-off synchrony of fields and units or the absence of unit activity despite well-defined seizure by field recording would seem to supersede the complex connectivity of the cerebral cortex. In terms of the dynamic pattern concept, this pattern appears to be a development of a new region of stability (albeit pathologic) owing to a change in the system parameters as a result of the application of an excess of ACh. This stability is manifested by the continuous clock-like recurrence of paroxysmal activity enduring for as long as one cares to observe it (Figure 75A). The paroxysms themselves, usually 1 to 3 sec long, and the interparoxysmal intervals of equal length constitute a complex pattern characterized by relatively sudden transitions, with onsets developing over 10 to 20 msec and offsets over 2 to 3 sec. These findings suggest the occurrence of system changes through an unstable transition separating two regions of relative stability for which the dynamic pattern model is proposed, akin to thresholds of the all-or-none type in which cooperativity dynamics operate. The term cooperativity implies an intended analogy of a sudden neuronal "bandwagon effect" to the biochemical cooperativity in nonMichaelis-Menten enzyme dynamics.

Ferguson also introduced evidence showing that a possible critical mass of neuronal generators may be necessary for the observed effects. This was indirectly demonstrated by the amount of cortical tissue needed, as measured from the edge of an ablated region, in order to demonstrate the paroxysmal activity described above. More distance, and therefore a greater mass of cortex, was needed for such a demonstration when measured from the edge of a large ablation than when measured from the edge of a smaller one. This again implies that a system property arises, depending on an adequate number and density of elements, and that it is comparatively independent of the basic properties of individual elements as they are observed in relative isolation.

Ferguson finds that the oscillatory patterns of the paroxysmal bursts are relatively unaffected by superficial lesions confined to the granular layer and above, but that the deep cortical negative shift is abolished by this intervention. He hypothesizes that loss of an inhibitory influence with the lesion abolishes the synchronizing of deep cortical cells that is necessary for the negative shift component. Presumably, this component is not essential for the maintenance of the new stability emerging from an ACh excess.

Prolonged Intracellular Depolarization: W. A. Spencer

Dichter and Spencer (1969a,b), using the deafferented fornix preparation (Spencer and Kandel, 1961c), detailed a study of penicillin-induced epileptic foci in the hippocampus, emphasizing the critical role of feedback circuitry in the genesis of interictal spikes (Ayala et al., 1973). Such behavior seems compatible with some of the dynamic pattern models referred to above (see the Appendix to Dichter and Spencer, 1969b, page 683).

Further study by Dichter and his co-workers (1972) demonstrated associated silent cell (presumed glial) depolarizations with a time course of many seconds (Figure 76). The onset of the depolari-

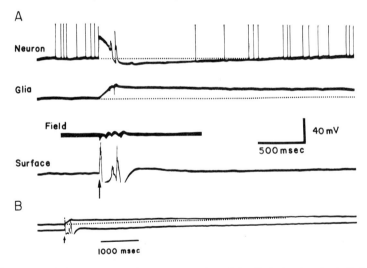

Figure 76. Intracellular responses of a neuron and a glial cell during interictal discharge. A. Intracellular recordings from a neuron and glial cell penetrated successively 100 μm apart. Both intracellular recordings occurred synchronously with the surface discharge. The "field" record is an extracellular potential recorded just below the neuron and above the glia. B. Same glial cell recording as in A but at a lower gain and slower sweep speed. Note the marked difference in time course of the depolarizations in the two cells. Positive is up in all traces. [Dichter et al., 1972]

zations was found to lag slightly behind that of neurons whose response coincides with the surface-recorded interictal spikes. Thus, the initial phase of the neuronal depolarization seems to depend on synaptic mechanisms; but the fact that prolonged silent cell depolarizations can summate when repeated stimuli are delivered some seconds apart raises the possibility that extracellular K^+ accumulation could play a significant role in the transition from isolated interictal spiking to sustained seizure activity. Studies of neocortical foci with K^+-sensitive micropipettes suggest similar K^+ accumulation dynamics (Prince et al., 1973).

Retinal Spreading Depression: A. Van Harreveld

Van Harreveld (1972) views the extracellular space (normally about 15% of the brain mass) as being dynamically maintained because it is sensitive to asphyxia and spreading depression with their concomitants of increased membrane permeability to Na^+ and to the movement of water and other extracellular material into cellular elements. The marked decrease in extracellular electrolytes is the basis of a noticeable increase in electrical impedance in these pathologic conditions. Van Harreveld speculates that changes of a similar kind, but to a lesser extent, occurring in the physiological range could lead to altered shapes of cellular elements and therefore of the dynamically maintained geometry of the extracellular space. Thus, the paths of currents flowing in the brain could also be altered. Whether such changes are of functional significance or whether they are epiphenomenal remains unknown.

Van Harreveld and Fifkova (1970) used the isolated chicken retina preparation of Martins-Ferreira and de Oliveira Castro (1966) that shows a sharp-edged, slowly advancing wave of increased transparency to light in association with the advancing front of spreading depression. They found that, at a threshold concentration of 0.2 mmole (a low value), glutamate triggers the retina to release labeled glutamate in good temporal correlation with the transparency change (Figure 77). They suggest that retinal release of glutamate by the application of a low concentration of the same compound is indicative of a positive feedback system underlying the all-or-none character of spreading depression. It may be possible to view this system in terms of a cooperativity or autocatalytic process brought to light in a relatively unphysiological way. Conceivably, the normal retina would have

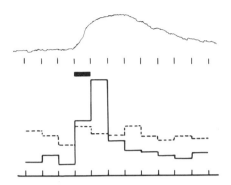

Figure 77. The upper line is a record of the transparency of the retinal tissue; an upward deflection indicates an enhanced transparency. Below this record the time is indicated in min. The bottom graphs represent histograms of the areas under the glutamate (solid lines) and glutamine (broken lines) peaks in the record of radioactivity in the 1-min samples of the fluid superfusing the retina charged with ^{14}C-glutamate. The bar indicates the 1-min application of a 0.5 mmole solution of unlabeled glutamate, after which the superfusion with the physiological salt solution was resumed. [Van Harreveld]

homeostatic constraints (whether passive or active) protecting it from the emergence of, or fostering its recovery from, such perturbations.

In contrast to glutamate, much higher relative concentrations of K^+ (threshold at 100 mmoles) are needed to trigger spreading depression. Van Harreveld and Fifkova (1973) observed that levels as low as 5 mmole of K^+ could induce a transparency change in the isolated chicken retina, but that 75 mmoles are required for the retina to release glutamate (Figure 78). Na^+ is required in the extracellular medium to provide the full transparency change. Moreover, it is the inward movement of this ion that is considered the key mechanism in the cellular swelling and changes in membrane position that underlie the altered light dispersion detected as increased transparency.

Mg^{2+} arrests spreading depression (Bureš, 1960) and Van Harreveld finds that, at a concentration of 10 to 15 mmoles, it blocks the transparency change in isolated retina; paradoxically, however, it does not block the release of glutamate. Propagating spreading depression can be elicited in the retina by locally applied KCl only in concentrations high enough to cause a release of glutamate, indicative of the central place of this amino acid in the process of propagation (Van Harreveld and Fifkova, 1973).

In Van Harreveld's opinion, different cellular elements can take up extracellular material under different conditions. For example, when K^+ concentrations as low as 5 mmoles are applied to neural tissue

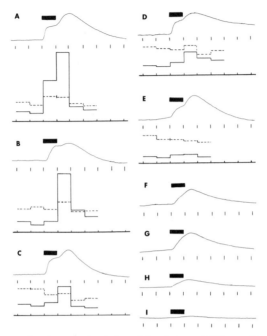

Figure 78. Responses of retinas to stimulation with solutions of different K⁺ concentrations. A to E. The upper parts of the figures show the records of the transparency change (an upward movement indicates increased transparency). The bar indicates the 1-min time signal. The lower parts of the figures show histograms of the areas under glutamine (broken lines) and glutamate (solid lines) peaks in the records of radioactivity of 1-min samples of the fluid superfusing the retina. F to I. Show only the transparency records since the stimulus did not cause a release of the label. The KCl concentration of the stimulating fluid in records A to I was 150, 125, 100, 75, 50, 30, 20, 10, and 5 mmoles, respectively, above the KCl concentration (3 mmoles) in the standard solution. [Van Harreveld and Fifkova, 1973]

cultures (Lodin et al., 1971), they cause an uptake of culture material and concomitantly, a swelling of the glial elements. By contrast, electron micrographs of the cortex during spreading depression (Van Harreveld and Khattab, 1967) show no glial swelling, but they do show swelling limited to dendritic elements, mainly the dendritic spines, which is postulated to be caused by a release of glutamate from the intracellular compartment.

V. IN RETROSPECT

Vernon Rowland

The core question of this Work Session report is: To what extent can progress in neuroscience be enhanced by awareness of and involvement with processes variously described as dynamic patterns, cooperative nonequilibrium phenomena, or dissipative structures? Aharon Katchalsky and Robert Blumenthal provided extensive reviews of the history and recent applications of the basic theme in physics, chemistry, and biology. For the most part, neuroscientists came to the Work Session having very little prior familiarity with the complexities underlying this theme. Furthermore, its direct applications to complex neuroscience problems are not readily apparent. The neuroscience applications at the Work Session are seen only as the earliest beginnings of a new field. Further assimilation than that attempted in this report of the neuroscience contributions in terms of the central theme is the task of future research.

A simplified view of the dynamic pattern concept is that it strives to describe accurately the mechanisms of emergence, of qualitative change suddenly appearing that cannot be reduced to a summation of quantitatively understood component processes. We may expect to penetrate, with dynamic pattern theory, the old aphorism stated here in the form of a question: What precisely is the difference that makes a whole (which is identified qualitatively) *more* than the sum of its quantitatively analyzed parts? The mystery is in the "more." The aphorism is practically a cliché used in expressing our ignorance of the mechanisms of emergence of life or of human awareness. If a whole is *less* than the sum of its parts, we can readily ascribe it to losses from competitive or interfering component processes. The "more," however, sounds like something for nothing, i.e., self-organizing systems arising out of unorganized soups; but Aharon Katchalsky directed our attention to the frequency of cooperative interactions in complex systems providing precisely the "more" that is needed to comprehend the "quality of the whole." It is not obtained for nothing, i.e., at no cost in energy, because the only systems displaying self-organizing dynamic patterns are those which dissipate energy in achieving and maintaining their self-organization. Similar thinking is implicit in such terms as synergy, in which the combined action of two chemical agents on a biological system is greater than the sum of their independent actions.

The neuroscience contributions of the participants at the Work Session neither unreservedly establish nor contradict the utility of dynamic pattern theory. The possibility of chemical waves, bulk oscillation, macrostates emerging out of cooperative processes, sudden transitions, prepatterning, etc., seem made to order to assist in the understanding of integrative processes, thresholds, synchronized actions, etc., of the nervous system—particularly in advancing questions of higher order functions that remain unexplained in terms of contemporary neurophysiology. But processes already established in neurophysiology are so rich in properties that adding dynamic pattern theory seems burdensome and superfluous rather than heuristic and simplifying. This is the challenge for future study of these matters.

It should be made explicit that true evaluation of the dynamic pattern theory can become derailed by issues that are transient and that arise during the familiarization process. An example of this developed at the Work Session and is preserved in the record in the issue of connectivity versus field actions (or as Freeman referred to it, as "oozism"). As these problems are worked through, it is to be hoped that the central enduring issues will be clarified. Is the propensity for dynamic patterning so intrinsic a property of complex nonequilibrium systems that to ignore it would be at great cost to progress in neuroscience? Is it so compelling a phenomenon that the nervous system can fail in bridling it and go through an unstable transition into a dramatic and pathologic dynamic pattern, the epileptic fit?

Hierarchical assembly of cooperative and competitive forces and flows depending on continuous energy dissipation is the only non-cosmic way we know that retards (never reverses) the unrelenting direction pointed by the second law of thermodynamics. Competitive forces and flows, in contrast to cooperative ones, were little considered at the Work Session, although emergent ideas were in competition among participants. As important as competition is for selection, it is only the prevailing of cooperative over competitive processes that leads to the survival of a pattern for us to perceive. Only this will guarantee the general survival of mankind.

ABBREVIATIONS

ACh	acetylcholine
cyclic AMP	adenosine-3',5'-phosphate
AEP	averaged evoked potential
CNV	contingent negative variation
CR	conditional response
CS	conditional stimulus
CSF	cerebrospinal fluid
ECoG	electrocorticogram
EEG	electroencephalogram
EOG	electrooculogram
EPSP	excitatory postsynaptic potential
FR	fixed ratio
FDP	fructose-1,6-diphosphate
F6P	fructose-6-phosphate
^{3}H-GABA	[^{3}H] γ-aminobutyric acid
GAP	glyceraldehyde-3-phosphate
IMU	integrated multiple unit activity
IPSP	inhibitory postsynaptic potential
NAD-NADH	nicotinamide adenine dinucleotide-reduced nicotinamide adenine dinucleotide
PSP	postsynaptic potential
PST	poststimulus time
SD	spreading depression
SP	steady potential
SPS	sustained potential shift
UCS	unconditional stimulus

154

BIBLIOGRAPHY

This bibliography contains two types of entries: (1) citations given or work alluded to in the report, and (2) additional references to pertinent literature by conference participants and others. Citations in group (1) may be found in the text on the pages in the right-hand column.

Page

Adey, W.R. (1967): Intrinsic organization of cerebral tissue in alerting, orienting, and discriminative responses. *In: The Neurosciences: A Study Program.* Quarton, G.C., Melnechuk, T., and Schmitt, F.O., eds. New York: Rockefeller University Press, pp. 615-633.

Adey, W.R. (1969): Slow electrical phenomena in the central nervous system.   80
Neurosciences Res. Prog. Bull. 7:75-180. Also *In: Neurosciences Research Symposium Summaries, Vol. 4.* Schmitt, F.O. et al., eds. Cambridge, Mass.: M.I.T. Press, 1970, pp. 1-102.

Adey, W.R. (1970): Spontaneous electrical brain rhythms accompanying learned responses. *In: The Neurosciences: Second Study Program.* Schmitt, F.O., editor-in-chief. New York: Rockefeller University Press, pp. 224-243.

Adey, W.R. (1971a): Cortical excitability changes following interaction of calcium   70,81,
with topical polyanions and glutamic acid. *Anat. Rec.* 169:265-266.   84

Adey, W.R. (1971b): Evidence for cerebral membrane effects of calcium, derived   80,81,
from direct-current gradient, impedance, and intracellular records. *Exp. Neurol.*   83
30:78-102.

Adey, W.R. (1972): Organization of brain tissue: is the brain a noisy processor? *Int. J. Neurosci.* 3:271-284.

Adey, W.R. (1974): The influences of impressed electrical fields at EEG frequencies   81
on brain and behavior. *In: Behavior and Brain Electrical Activity.* Altshuler, H. and Burch, N.R., eds. New York: Plenum Press. (In press)

Adey, W.R. and Baker, M.A. (1972): Temperature effects on membrane potentials of cortical neurons in cat. *Fed. Proc.* 31:303. (Abstr.)

Adey, W.R., Bystrom, B.G., Costin, A., Kado, R.T., and Tarby, T.J. (1969):   80
Divalent cations in cerebral impedance and cell membrane morphology. *Exp. Neurol.* 23:29-50.

Adey, W.R., Kado, R.T., and Didio, J. (1962): Impedance measurements in brain tissue of animals using microvolt signals. *Exp. Neurol.* 5:47-66.

Adey, W.R., Walter, D.O., and Hendrix, C.E. (1961): Computer techniques in correlation and spectral analyses of cerebral slow waves during discriminative behavior. *Exp. Neurol.* 3:501-524.

Ahmed, N. and Van Harreveld, A. (1969): The iodide space in rabbit brain. *J. Physiol.* 204:31-50.

Page

Aladjalova, N.A. (1964): *Slow Electrical Processes in the Brain. Progress in Brain Research, Vol. 7.* Amsterdam: Elsevier.
63

Anand, J.N. and Balwinski, R.Z. (1969): Surface deformation of thin coatings caused by evaporative convection. I. Macroscopic surface replication. *J. Colloid Interf. Sci.* 31:196-202.
17

Andersen, P. and Andersson, S. (1968): *Physiological Basis of the Alpha Rhythm.* New York: Appleton-Century-Crofts, Inc.
109

Andersen, P. and Eccles, J.C. (1962): Inhibitory phasing of neuronal discharge. *Nature* 196:645-647.
108

Andersen, P., Eccles, J.C., and Loyning, Y. (1964): Pathway of postsynaptic inhibition in the hippocampus. *J. Neurophysiol.* 27:608-619.
108

Andersen, P., Gillow, M., and Rudjord, T. (1966): Rhythmic activity in a simulated neuronal network. *J. Physiol.* 185:418-428.

Anderson, P.W. (1972): More is different. Broken symmetry and the nature of the hierarchical structure of science. *Science* 177:393-396.
21

Anderson, R. and Rowland, V. (1971): Brain steady potential shifts. *In: Progress in Physiological Psychology, Vol. 4.* Stellar, E. and Sprague, J.M., eds. New York: Academic Press, pp. 37-51.

Anninos, P.A. (1972a): Cyclic modes in artificial neural nets. *Kybernetik* 11:5-14.
101

Anninos, P.A. (1972b): Mathematical model of memory trace and forgetfulness. *Kybernetik* 10:165-167.
99

Anninos, P.A., Beek, B., Csermely, T.J., Harth, E.M., and Pertile, G. (1970): Dynamics of neural structures. *J. Theor. Biol.* 26:121-148.
99

Anninos, P.A. and Elul, R. (1971): Dynamic changes in inter-neuronal coupling in artificial nerve nets. *Biophysical Society Abstracts.* Fifteenth Annual Meeting, New Orleans, La. 11:242a.

Anninos, P. and Elul, R. (1972): A neural net model for the alpha-rhythm. *Biophysical Society Abstracts.* Sixteenth Annual Meeting, Toronto, Canada. 12:267a.

Anninos, P.A. and Elul, R. (1972): Relationship of anatomy and function in CNS: a neuronal model study. *In: Program and Abstracts, Society for Neuroscience.* Second Annual Meeting, Houston, Tex., p. 256.

Arduini, A.A. (1958): Enduring potential changes evoked in the cerebral cortex by stimulation of brain stem reticular formation and thalamus. *In: Reticular Formation of the Brain.* Jasper, H.H. et al., eds. Boston: Little, Brown and Co., pp. 333-351.
127

Arvanitaki, A. (1942): Effects evoked in an axon by the activity of a contiguous one. *J. Neurophysiol.* 5:89-108.
138

156

Asahina, K. and Yamanaka, M. (1960): The relationship between steady potential and other electrical activities of cerebral cortex. *Jap. J. Physiol.* 10:258-266.

Aschoff, J. (1965): Circadian rhythms in man. *Science* 148:1427-1432. 71

Attneave, F. (1971): Multistability in perception. *Sci. Am.* 225:63-71. 12

Avsec, D. (1939): Tourbillon thermoconvectifs dans l'air application à la météorologie. *Public. Sci. Techn. Minist. Air* (Paris) 155:1-214. 15

Ayala, G.F., Dichter, M., Gumnit, R.J., Matsumoto, H., and Spencer, W.A. (1973): Genesis of epileptic interictal spikes. New knowledge of cortical feedback systems suggests a neurophysiological explanation of brief paroxysms. *Brain Res.* 52:1-17. 147

Bahng, J. and Schwarzschild, M. (1961): Lifetime of solar granules. *Astrophys. J.* 134:312-322. 21

Baker, R. and Llinás, R. (1971): Electrotonic coupling between neurones in the rat mesencephalic nucleus. *J. Physiol.* 212:45-63.

Bangham, A.D. and Horne, R.W. (1962): Action of saponin on biological cell membranes. *Nature* 196:952-953. 17,18

Barlow, H.B. and Pettigrew, J.D. (1971): Lack of specificity of neurones in the visual cortex of young kittens. *J. Physiol.* 218:98P-100P.

Bawin, S.M., Gavalas-Medidi, R.J., and Adey, W.R. (1973): Effects of modulated very high frequency fields on specific brain rhythms in cats. *Brain Res.* 58:365-384. 140,142

Beck, M.T. and Váradi, Z.B. (1972): One, two and three-dimensional spatially periodic chemical reactions. *Nature Phys. Sci.* 235:15-16. 56

Becker, J.-U. and Betz, A. (1972): Membrane transport as controlling pacemaker of glycolysis in *Saccharomyces carlsbergensis*. *Biochim. Biophys. Acta* 274:584-597. 70

Beidler, L.M. (1954): Physiological problems in odor research. *Ann. N.Y. Acad. Sci.* 58:52-57.

Belousov, B.P. (1958): Sborn referat. radiat. meditsin za. *In: Collection of Abstracts on Radiation Medicine.* Moscow: Medgiz, 1959, p. 145. 30

Bénard, H. (1901): Les tourbillons cellulaires dans une nappe liquide transportant de la chaleur par convection en régime permanent. *Ann. Chim. Phys.* 23:62-144. 12

Bennett, M.V.L. (1966): Physiology of electrotonic junctions. *Ann. N.Y. Acad. Sci.* 137:509-539. 90

Bennett, M.V.L. (1971): Electrolocation in fish. *Ann. N.Y. Acad. Sci.* 188:242-269.

Bennett, M.V.L. (1972a): A comparison of electrically and chemically mediated   90
transmission. *In: Structure and Function of Synapses.* Pappas, G.D. and Purpura,
D.P., eds. New York: Raven Press, pp. 221-256.

Bennett, M.V.L. (1972b): Electrical versus chemical neurotransmission. *In:*   90
Neurotransmitters. Kopin, I.J., ed. Baltimore: Williams and Wilkins, pp. 58-90.

Bennett, M.V.L. (1973): Function of electrotonic junctions in embryonic and adult
tissues. *Fed. Proc.* 32:65-75.

Bennett, M.V.L. and Auerbach, A.A. (1969): Calculation of electrical coupling of   87
cells separated by a gap. *Anat. Rec.* 163:152. (Abstr.)

Bennett, M.V.L. and Spira, M.E. (1971): Properties of junctions mediating
electrical coupling between embryonic cells. *Biol. Bull.* 141:378.

Bennett, M.V.L., Spira, M.E., and Pappas, G.D. (1972): Properties of electrotonic
junctions between embryonic cells of *Fundulus. Dev. Biol.* 29:419-435.

Bernal, J.D. (1951): *The Physical Basis of Life.* London: Routledge and Paul.   45

Bernal, J.D. (1967): *Origin of Life.* New York: Universe Books.

Bernhard, C.G. (1958): On undifferentiated neuronal spread of excitation. *Exp.*   138
Cell Res. 5(Suppl.):201-220.

Betz, A. and Chance, B. (1965): Phase relationship of glycolytic intermediates in   70
yeast cells with oscillatory metabolic control. *Arch. Biochem. Biophys.*
109:585-594.

Beurle, R.L. (1956): Properties of a mass of cells capable of regenerating pulses.   73,74
Phil. Trans. Roy. Soc. B 240:55-94.

Biedenbach, M.A. and Freeman, W.J. (1965): Linear domain of potentials from the
prepyriform cortex with respect to stimulus parameters. *Exp. Neurol.*
11:400-417.

Bindman, L.J., Lippold, O.C., and Redfearn, J.W.T. (1962): Long-lasting changes in
the level of the electrical activity of the cerebral cortex produced by polarizing
currents. *Nature* 196:584-585.

Bishop, G.H. and O'Leary, J.L. (1950): The effects of polarizing currents on cell
potentials and their significance in the interpretation of central nervous activity.
Electroencephalogr. Clin. Neurophysiol. 2:401-416.

Blakemore, C., Carpenter, R.H.S., and Georgeson, M.A. (1970): Lateral inhibition
between orientation detectors in the human visual system. *Nature* 228:37-39.

Blakemore, C., Carpenter, R.H.S., and Georgeson, M.A. (1971): Lateral thinking
about lateral inhibition. *Nature* 234:418-419.

Blakemore, C. and Cooper, G.F. (1970): Development of the brain depends on the
visual environment. *Nature* 228:477-478.

158

Blakemore, C. and Mitchell, D.E. (1973): Environmental modification of the visual cortex and the neural basis of learning and memory. *Nature* 241:467-468.

Blakemore, C. and Tobin, E.A. (1972): Lateral inhibition between orientation detectors in the cat's visual cortex. *Exp. Brain Res.* 15:439-440.

Blakemore, C. and Van Sluyters, R.C. (1974): Reversal of the physiological effects of monocular deprivation in the kitten: further evidence for a sensitive period. *J. Physiol.* (In press)

Blumenthal, R.P. (1973): Dynamic patterns in active transport. *Isr. J. Chem.* 11:341-355.   67,70

Blumenthal, R., Changeux, J.-P., and Lefever, R. (1970): Membrane excitability and dissipative instabilities. *J. Membr. Biol.* 2:351-374.   54,65, 66,67

Bonhoeffer, K.F. (1948): Activation of passive iron as a model for the excitation of nerve. *J. Gen. Physiol.* 32:69-91.   34

Bonhoeffer, K.F. (1953): Modelle der Nervenerregung. *Naturwissenschaften* 40:301-311.   34,57

Bonner, J.T. (1967): *The Cellular Slime Molds.* 2nd Ed. Princeton, N.J.: Princeton University Press.

Bonner, J.T., Barkley, D.S., Hall, E.M., Konijn, T.M., Mason, J.W., O'Keefe, G., III, and Wolfe, P.B. (1969): Acrasin, acrasinase, and the sensitivity to acrasin in *Dictyostelium discoideum. Dev. Biol.* 20:72-87.   50

Bourke, R.S., Nelson, K.M., Naumann, R.A., and Young, O.M. (1970): Studies of the production and subsequent reduction of swelling in primate cerebral cortex under isosmotic conditions in vivo. *Exp. Brain Res.* 10:427-446.   128

Bricker, N.S., Biber, T., and Ussing, H.H. (1963): Exposure of the isolated frog skin to high potassium concentrations at the internal surface. I. Bioelectric phenomena and sodium transport. *J. Clin. Invest.* 42:88-99.   127

Brookhart, J.M. and Blachly, P.H. (1952): Cerebellar unit responses to DC polarization. *Am. J. Physiol.* 171:711. (Abstr.)

Brookhart, J.M. and Kubota, K. (1963): Studies of the integrative function of the motor neurone. *Prog. Brain Res.* 1:38-64.

Bruce, V.G. (1960): Environmental entrainment of circadian rhythms. *Cold Spring Harbor Symp. Quant. Biol.* 25:29-48.   71

Brunt, D. (1937): Natural and artificial clouds. *Q. J. Roy. Meteorol. Soc.* 63:277-288.   20

Buck, J. and Buck, E. (1966): Biology of synchronous flashing of fireflies. *Nature* 211:562-564.   71

Bullock, T.H. (1959): Neuron doctrine and electrophysiology. *Science* 129:997-1002.

Bullock, T.H. (1966): Integrative properties of neural tissue. *In: Frontiers in Physiological Psychology.* New York: Academic Press, pp. 5-20.

Bullock, T.H. (1974): Comparisons between vertebrates and invertebrates in nervous organization. *In: The Neurosciences: Third Study Program.* Schmitt, F.O. and Worden, F.G., eds. Cambridge, Mass.: M.I.T. Press, pp. 343-346.   95

Bullock, T.H. and Horridge, G.A. (1965): *Structure and Function in The Nervous*   71,72,
Systems of Invertebrates, Vol. I. San Francisco: W.H. Freeman, p. 461.   73

Bureš, J. (1957): The ontogenetic development of steady potential differences in the cerebral cortex in animals. *Electroencephalogr. Clin. Neurophysiol.* 9:121-130.

Bureš, J. (1959): Reversible decortication and behavior. *In: The Central Nervous System and Behavior.* Brazier, M.A.B., ed. New York: Josiah Macy, Jr. Foundation, pp. 207-248.

Bureš, J. (1960): Block of Leão's spreading cortical depression by bivalent cations.   149
Physiol. Bohemoslov. 9:202-209.

Bureš, J. and Burešová, O. (1956): The question of ionic antagonism in spreading depression. *Physiol. Bohemoslov.* 5:195-205.

Bureš, J. and Burešová, O. (1960): The use of Leão's spreading cortical depression   127
in research on conditioned reflexes. *In: The Moscow Colloquium on Electroencephalography of Higher Nervous Activity.* Jasper, H.H. and Smirnov, G.D., eds. *Electroencephalogr. Clin. Neurophysiol.* 13(Suppl.):359-376.

Bureš, J. and Burešová, O. (1967): Plastic changes of unit activity based on reinforcing properties of extracellular stimulation of single neurons. *J. Neurophysiol.* 30:98-113.

Bureš, J., Burešová, O., and Záhorová, A. (1958): Conditioned reflexes and Leão's spreading cortical depression. *J. Comp. Physiol. Psychol.* 51:263-268.

Burns, B.D. (1954): The production of after-bursts in isolated unanesthetized cerebral cortex. *J. Physiol.* 125:427-446.

Burns, B.D. (1955): The mechanism of after-bursts in cerebral cortex. *J. Physiol.* 127:168-188.

Burton, A.C. (1939): The properties of the steady state compared to those of   27
equilibrium as shown in characteristic biological behavior. *J. Cell. Comp. Physiol.* 14:327-349.

Busse, F.H. and Whitehead, J.A. (1971): Instabilities of convection rolls in a high Prandtl number fluid. *J. Fluid Mech.* 47:305-320.

Busse, H.G. (1969): A spatial periodic homogeneous chemical reaction. *J. Phys.*   31,32
Chem. 73:750.

160

Calvet, J., Calvet, M.C., and Scherrer, J. (1964): Étude stratigraphique corticale de l'activité EEG spontanée. *Electroencephalogr. Clin. Neurophysiol.* 17:109-125.

Calvet, J. and Scherrer, J. (1961): Relation des décharges unitaires avec les ondes cérébrales spontanées et la polarization corticale. *C. R. Acad. Sci.* 252: 2297-2299.

Castellucci, V.F. and Goldring, S. (1970): Contribution to steady potential shifts of slow depolarization in cells presumed to be glia. *Electroencephalogr. Clin. Neurophysiol.* 28:109-118.   121

Chance, B., Estabrook, R.W., and Ghosh, A. (1964): Damped sinusoidal oscillations of cytoplasmic reduced pyridine nucleotide in yeast cells. *Proc. Nat. Acad. Sci.* 51:1244-1251.   60,62

Chance, B., Estabrook, R.W., and Williamson, J.R., eds. (1965): *Control of Energy Metabolism.* New York: Academic Press.   60

Chandrasekhar, S. (1961): *Hydrodynamic and Hydromagnetic Stability.* New York: Oxford University Press.

Changeux, J.-P. (1966): Responses of acetylcholinesterase from *Torpedo marmorata* to salts and curarizing drugs. *Mol. Pharmacol.* 2:369-392.   65

Changeux, J.-P. (1969): Symmetry and function of biological systems at the macromolecular level. *In: Nobel Symposium No. 11.* Engström, A. and Strandberg, B., eds. New York: John Wiley and Sons, Inc., p. 235.   65,66

Changeux, J.-P. and Podleski, T.R. (1968): On the excitability and cooperativity of the electroplax membrane. *Proc. Nat. Acad. Sci.* 59:944-950.   65

Changeux, J.-P. and Thiéry, J. (1968): On the excitability and cooperativity of biological membranes. *In: Regulatory Functions of Biological Membranes.* Järnefelt, J., ed. Amsterdam: Elsevier, pp. 116-138.   65

Changeux, J.-P., Thiéry, J., Tung, Y., and Kittel, C. (1967): On the cooperativity of biological membranes. *Proc. Nat. Acad. Sci.* 57:335-341.   66

Clark, L.C., Jr. and Mishrahy, G. (1957): Chronically implanted polarograph electrodes. *Fed. Proc.* 16:22. (Abstr.)   63

Clark, L.C., Jr. and Sachs, G. (1968): Bioelectrodes for tissue metabolism. *Ann. N.Y. Acad. Sci.* 148:133-153.   63

Cohen, D. (1972): Magnetoencephalography: detection of the brain's electrical activity with a superconducting magnetometer. *Science* 175:664-666.

Cohen, M.W. (1970): The contribution by glial cells to surface recordings from the optic nerve of an amphibian. *J. Physiol.* 210:565-580.

Cole, K.S. (1968): *Membranes, Ions and Impulses.* Berkeley: University of California Press.   67

Collewijn, H. and Van Harreveld, A. (1966): Membrane potential of cerebral cortical cells during spreading depression and asphyxia. *Exp. Neurol.* 15:425-436.

Costin, A., Bystrom, B., Rovner, E., and Sabbot, I. (1974): Effect of a chelating ion exchange resin (Chelex 100) on impedance and evoked potentials. *Experientia.* (In press)

84

Cowan, J. (1970): Statistical mechanics of neural nets. *In: Mathematical Questions in the Life Sciences, Vol. 2.* Gerstenhaber, M., ed. Providence, R.I.: American Mathematical Society.

56

Cowley, M.D. and Rosensweig, R.E. (1967): The interfacial stability of a ferromagnetic fluid. *J. Fluid Mech.* 30:671-688.

19

Crain, S.M. and Bornstein, M.B. (1972): Organotypic bioelectric activity in cultured reaggregates of dissociated rodent brain cells. *Science* 176:182-184.

Creutzfeldt, O.D., Fromm, G.H., and Kapp, H. (1962): Influence of transcortical d-c currents on cortical neuronal activity. *Exp. Neurol.* 5:436-452.

132

Creutzfeldt, O.D., Watanabe, S., and Lux, H.D. (1966a): Relations between EEG phenomena and potentials of single cortical cells. I. Evoked responses after thalamic and epicortical stimulation. *Electroencephalogr. Clin. Neurophysiol.* 20:1-18.

Creutzfeldt, O.D., Watanabe, S., and Lux, H.D. (1966b): Relations between EEG phenomena and potentials of single cortical cells. II. Spontaneous and convulsoid activity. *Electroencephalogr. Clin. Neurophysiol.* 20:19-37.

Cuatrecasas, P. (1971): Insulin-receptor interactions in adipose tissue cells: direct measurement and properties. *Proc. Nat. Acad. Sci.* 68:1264-1268.

144

Davies, P.W. and Bronk, D.W. (1957): Oxygen tension in mammalian brain. *Fed. Proc.* 16:689-692.

63

Degn, H. (1972): Oscillating chemical reactions in homogeneous phase. *J. Chem. Educ.* 49:302-307.

30

DeHaan, R.L. (1967): Introduction: spontaneous activity of cultured heart cells. *In: Factors Influencing Myocardial Contractility.* Tanz, R.D., Kavaler, F., and Roberts, J., eds. New York: Academic Press, pp. 217-230.

72

DeHaan, R.L. (1968): Emergence of form and function in the embryonic heart. *Dev. Biol.* 2(Suppl.):208-250.

DeHaan, R.L. and Sachs, H.G. (1972): Cell coupling in developing systems: the heart-cell paradigm. *Curr. Top. Dev. Biol.* 7:193-228.

60,64, 72

Denny, D. and Brookhart, J.M. (1962): The effects of applied polarization on evoked electro-cortical waves in the cat. *Electroencephalogr. Clin. Neurophysiol.* 14:885-897.

162

Page

DeSimone, J.A., Beil, D.L., Scriven, L.E. (1973): Ferroin-collodion membranes: 33
dynamic concentration patterns in planar membranes. *Science* 180:946-949.

Deza, L. and Eidelberg, E. (1967): Development of cortical electrical activity in the 127
rat. *Exp. Neurol.* 17:425-438.

Dichter, M.A., Herman, C.J., and Selzer, M. (1972): Silent cells during interictal 109,147
discharges and seizures in hippocampal penicillin foci. Evidence for the role of
extracellular K^+ in the transition from the interictal state to seizures. *Brain Res.*
48:113-183.

Dichter, M. and Spencer, W.A. (1969a): Penicillin-induced interictal discharges 147
from the cat hippocampus: I. Characteristics and topographical features.
J. Neurophysiol. 32:649-662.

Dichter, M. and Spencer, W.A. (1969b): Penicillin-induced interictal discharges 147
from the cat hippocampus: II. Mechanisms underlying origin and restriction.
J. Neurophysiol. 32:663-687.

Diels, H. (1909): *Herakleitos von Ephesos.* (Greek and German) 2nd Ed. Berlin. 11

Donchin, E., Gerbrandt, L.A., Leifer, L., and Tucker, L. (1972): Is the contingent
negative variation contingent on a motor response? *Psychophysiology*
9:178-188.

Donchin, E., Otto, D., Gerbrandt, L.K., and Pribram, K.H. (1971): While a monkey
waits: electrocortical events recorded during the foreperiod of a reaction time
study. *Electroencephalogr. Clin. Neurophysiol.* 31:115-127.

Dourmashkin, R.R., Dougherty, R.M., and Harris, J.C. (1962): Electron micro- 17
scopic observations on rous sarcoma virus and cell membranes. *Nature*
194:1116-1119.

Eccles, J.C., Kostyuk, P.G., and Schmidt, R.F. (1962): The effect of electric
polarization of the spinal cord on central afferent fibres and on their excitatory
synaptic action. *J. Physiol.* 162:138-150.

Ehrenstein, G., Lecar, H., and Nossal, R. (1970): The nature of the negative
resistance in bimolecular lipid membranes containing excitability-inducing
material. *J. Gen. Physiol.* 55:119-133.

Eidelberg, E. (1962): Cortical steady potentials. A discussion of some possible 82,127
mechanisms for their production. *Bol. Inst. Estud. Méd. Biol., Méx.* 20:221-231.

Eidelberg, E. (1963): Cortical steady potential dependence on ionic environment. 82
Physiologist 6:175.

Eidelberg, E., Kolmodin, G.M., and Meyerson, B.A. (1965): Ontogenesis of steady 127
potential and direct cortical response in fetal sheep brain. *Exp. Neurol.*
12:198-214.

Eidelberg, E., Kolmodin, G.M., and Meyerson, B.A. (1967): Effect of asphyxia on
the cortical steady potential in adult and fetal sheep. *Acta Physiol. Scand.*
69:257-261.

Eidelberg, E. and Meyerson, B.A. (1964): Effects of lidocaine on cortical dendritic activity. *Arch. Int. Pharmacodyn.* 147:576-585.

Eigen, M. (1971a): Molecular self-organization and the early stages of evolution. *Q. Rev. Biophys.* 4:149-212.   46,48

Eigen, M. (1971b): Selforganization of matter and the evolution of biological macromolecules. *Naturwissenschaften* 58:465-523.

Eigen, M. (1974): Molecules, information, and memory: from molecular to neural   48
networks. *In: The Neurosciences: Third Study Program.* Schmitt, F.O. and
Worden, F.G., eds. Cambridge, Mass.: M.I.T. Press, pp. xix-xxvii.

Elul, R. (1966): Applications of non-uniform electric fields. Part 1. Electrophoretic
evaluation of adsorption. *Faraday Soc. Trans.*, pp. 3484-3492.

Elul, R. (1968): Brain waves: intracellular recording and statistical analysis help   97
clarify their physiological significance. *In: Data Acquisition and Processing in
Biology and Medicine, Vol. V.* Enslein, K., ed. New York: Pergamon Press,
pp. 93-115.

Elul, R. (1969a): Gaussian behavior of the electroencephalogram: changes during
performance of mental task. *Science* 164:328-331.

Elul, R. (1969b): Spatial organization of synaptic inputs to neurons in cerebral
cortex. *Biophysical Society Abstracts.* Thirteenth Annual Meeting, Los Angeles,
Calif. 9:64a.

Elul, R. (1972a): The genesis of the EEG. *Int. Rev. Neurobiol.* 15:227-272.   98

Elul, R. (1972b): Randomness and synchrony in the generation of the electro-   98
encephalogram. *In: Synchronization of EEG Activity in Epilepsies.* Petsche, H.
and Brazier, M.A.B., eds. New York: Springer-Verlag, pp. 59-77.

Emery, J.D. and Freeman, W.J. (1969): Pattern analysis of cortical evoked
potential parameters during attention changes. *Physiol. Behav.* 4:69-77.

Fatt, P. (1957): Electric potentials occurring around a neurone during its   137
antidromic activation. *J. Neurophysiol.* 20:27-60.

Fehmi, L.G. and Bullock, T.H. (1967): Discrimination among temporal patterns of   73
stimulation in a computer model of a coelenterate nerve net. *Kybernetik*
3:240-249.

Feldman, M.H. and Goldring, S. (1969): Osmotically induced changes in brain
steady potential and auditory evoked response. *Electroencephalogr. Clin.
Neurophysiol.* 26:588-596.

Feldman, M.H. and Purpura, D.P. (1970): Prolonged conductance increase in
thalamic neurons during synchronizing inhibition. *Brain Res.* 24:329-332.

Ferguson, J.H. (1972a): The effect of cortical laminar thermocoagulation on   145
epileptiform DC shift. *Neurology* 22:412. (Abstr.)

Page

Ferguson, J.H. (1972b): Laminar DC analysis of acetylcholine-induced epileptiform   145
activity in chronically undercut cortex. *Epilepsia* 13:352-353. (Abstr.)

Ferguson, J.H. and Cornblath, D.R. (1974): Acetylcholine epilepsy: modification   145
of DC shift in chronically undercut cat cortex. *Electroencephalogr. Clin.
Neurophysiol.* (In press)

Ferguson, J.H., Cornblath, D.R., and Havre, P.A. (1973): Determination of critical
mass for acetylcholine induced seizure activity. *In: Program and Abstracts,
Society for Neuroscience.* Third Annual Meeting, San Diego, Calif., p. 198.

Ferguson, J.H. and Jasper, H.H. (1971): Laminar DC studies of acetylcholine-   145
activated epileptiform discharge in cerebral cortex. *Electroencephalogr. Clin.
Neurophysiol.* 30:377-390.

Fertziger, A.P. and Purpura, D.P. (1971): Diphasic-PSPs during maintained activity
of cat lateral geniculate neurons. *Brain Res.* 33:463-467.

Field, R.J. (1972): A reaction periodic in time and space. *J. Chem. Educ.*   31
49:308-311.

Fifková, E. and Syka, J. (1964): Relationships between cortical and striatal
spreading depression in rat. *Exp. Neurol.* 9:355-366.

Fifková, E. and Van Harreveld, A. (1970): Glutamatè effects in the developing
chicken. *Exp. Neurol.* 28:286-298.

Finlayson, B.A. and Scriven, L.E. (1966): On the search for variational principles.
Int. J. Heat Mass Transfer 10:799-821.

FitzHugh, R. (1961): Impulses and physiological states in theoretical models of   27,29
nerve membrane. *Biophys. J.* 1:445-466.

FitzHugh, R. (1969): Mathematical models of excitation and propagation in nerve.   24,27,
In: Biological Engineering. Schwan, H.P., ed. New York: McGraw-Hill, pp. 1-85.   29

Fox, S.W. (1965): A theory of macromolecular and cellular origins. *Nature*
205:328-340.

Freeman, W.J. (1963): The electrical activity of a primary sensory cortex: analysis
of EEG waves. *Int. Rev. Neurobiol.* 5:53-119.

Freeman, W.J. (1964): A linear distributed feedback model for prepyriform cortex.
Exp. Neurol. 10:525-547.

Freeman, W.J. (1964): Use of digital adaptive filters for measuring prepyriform
evoked potentials from cats. *Exp. Neurol.* 10:475-492.

Freeman, W.J. (1967): Analysis of function of cerebral cortex by use of control   76
systems theory. *Logistics Rev.* 3(12):5-40.

Freeman, W.J. (1968a): Analog stimulation of prepyriform cortex in the cat. *Math.
Biosci.* 2:181-190.

Freeman, W.J. (1968b): Patterns of variation in waveform of averaged evoked potentials from prepyriform cortex of cats. *J. Neurophysiol.* 31:1-13.

Freeman, W.J. (1968c): Relations between unit activity and evoked potentials in prepyriform cortex of cats. *J. Neurophysiol.* 31:337-348.

Freeman, W.J. (1968d): Effects of surgical isolation and tetanization on prepyriform cortex in cats. *J. Neurophysiol.* 31:349-357.   76

Freeman, W.J. (1970): Amplitude and excitability changes of prepyriform cortex related to work performance by cats. *J. Biomed. Systems* 1:23-29.

Freeman, W.J. (1970): Spectral analysis of prepyriform averaged evoked potentials in cats. *J. Biomed. Systems* 1:3-22.

Freeman, W.J. (1972a): Spatial divergence and temporal dispersion in primary   101,105
olfactory nerve of cat. *J. Neurophysiol.* 35:733-744.

Freeman, W.J. (1972b): Measurement of open loop responses to electrical   101
stimulation in olfactory bulb of cat. *J. Neurophysiol.* 35:745-761.

Freeman, W.J. (1972c): Measurement of oscillatory responses to electrical   101,105
stimulation in olfactory bulb of cat. *J. Neurophysiol.* 35:762-779.

Freeman, W.J. (1972d): Depth recording of averaged evoked potential of olfactory   101
bulb. *J. Neurophysiol.* 35:780-796.

Freeman, W.J. (1972e): Linear analysis of the dynamics of neural masses. *Annu.*   101
Rev. Biophys. Bioeng. 1:225-256.

Freeman, W.J. (1972f): Wave transmission by olfactory neurons. *Fed. Proc.*   101
31:855. (Abstr.)

Freeman, W.J. (1972g): Waves, pulses and the theory of neural masses. *Prog. Theor.*   101,103,
Biol. 2:88-165.   105,106

Freeman, W.J. (1973a): Attenuation of transmission through glomeruli of olfactory bulb on paired shock stimulation. *Brain Res.* 65:77-90.

Freeman, W.J. (1973b): A model of the olfactory system. *In: Neural Modeling*   104
(Brain Information Service Research Report No. 1). Brazier, M.A.B., Walter, D.O., and Schneider, D., eds. Los Angeles: Brain Research Institute, University of California at Los Angeles, pp. 41-62.

Freeman, W.J. (1973c): Relation of glomerular neuronal activity to glomerular   104
transmission attenuation. *Brain Res.* 65:91-107.

Fromm, G.H. and Glass, J.D. (1970): Influence of cortical steady potential on evoked potentials and neuron activity. *Exp. Neurol.* 27:426-437.

Fuortes, M.G.F. (1954): Direct current stimulation of motoneurons. *J. Physiol.* 126:494-506.

Page

Gavalas, R.J., Walter, D.O., Hamer, J., and Adey, W.R. (1970): Effect of low-level, low-frequency electric fields on EEG and behavior in *Macaca nemestrina*. *Brain Res.* 18:491-501.
140,141, 142

Gerard, R.W. (1942): Electrophysiology. *Annu. Rev. Physiol.* 4:329-358.
87

Gerisch, G. (1972): Oscillations as a basis of spatial patterns in cellular slime molds. *In: Genesis of Neuronal Patterns.* Edds, M.E., Barkley, D.S., and Fambrough, D.M. *Neurosciences Res. Prog. Bull.* 10:326-330.
57

Gessi, T. (1971): Multiple collateral pathways in hippocampus. *Proc. Int. Union Physiol. Sci.* 9:201. (Abstr.)
107,108

Gijsbers, K.J. and Melzack, R. (1967): Oxygen tension changes evoked in the brain by visual stimulation. *Science* 156:1392-1393.
63

Glansdorff, P., Nicolis, G., and Prigogine, I. (1974): The thermodynamic stability theory of non-equilibrium states. *Proc. Nat. Acad. Sci.* 71:197-199.
42

Glansdorff, P. and Prigogine, I. (1971): *Thermodynamic Theory of Structure, Stability and Fluctuations.* New York: Wiley-Interscience.
46,76

Glauert, A.M., Dingle, J.T., and Lucy, J.A. (1962): Action of saponin on biological membranes. *Nature* 196:953-955.
18

Gmitro, J.L. and Scriven, L.E. (1966): A physicochemical basis for pattern and rhythm. *In: Intracellular Transport.* Warren, K.B., ed. New York: Academic Press, pp. 221-255.
13,36, 37,38, 57,58

Goldbeter, A. and Lefever, R. (1972): Dissipative structures for an allosteric model. Application to glycolytic oscillations. *Biophys. J.* 12:1302-1315.
62

Goodenough, D.A. and Stoeckenius, W. (1972): The isolation of mouse hepatocyte gap junctions. Preliminary chemical characterization and X-ray diffraction. *J. Cell Biol.* 54:646-656.
91

Goodwin, B.C. (1963): *The Temporal Organization in Cells.* New York: Academic Press.
55,56

Goodwin, B.C. and Cohen, M.H. (1969): A phase-shift model for the spatial and temporal organization of developing systems. *J. Theor. Biol.* 25:49-107.
42,65

Gorman, A.L.F. (1966): Differential patterns of activation of the pyramidal system elicited by surface anodal and cathodal cortical stimulation. *J. Neurophysiol.* 29:547-564.

Grafstein, B. (1956): Mechanisms of spreading cortical depression. *J. Neurophysiol.* 19:154-171.
127

Granit, R., Kernall, D., and Smith, R.S. (1963): Delayed depolarization and the repetitive response to intracellular stimulation of mammalian motoneurones. *J. Physiol.* 168:890-910.

Granit, R. and Phillips, C.G. (1957): Effects on Purkinje cells of surface stimulation of the cerebellum. *J. Physiol.* 135:73-92.

Granit, R. and Skoglund, C.R. (1945): Facilitation, inhibition and depression at the "artificial synapse" formed by the cut end of a mammalian nerve. *J. Physiol.* 103:435-448.   138

Gray, E.G. (1961): The granule cells, mossy synapses and Purkinje spine synapses of the cerebellum: light and electron microscope observations. *J. Anat.* 95:345-356.   87

Grobstein, P., Chow, K.L., Spear, P.D., and Mathers, L.H. (1973): Development of rabbit visual cortex: late appearance of a class of receptive fields. *Science* 180:1185-1187.

Grossman, R.G. (1972a): Alterations in the microphysiology of glial cells and neurons and their environment in injured brain. *Clin. Neurosurg.* 19:69-83.   132

Grossman, R.G. (1972b): The glia. *In: Scientific Foundations of Neurology.* Critchley, M., O'Leary, J.L., and Jennett, B., eds. Philadelphia: F.A. Davis Co., pp. 9-21.   129

Grossman, R.G. and Rosman, L.J. (1971): Intracellular potentials of inexcitable cells in epileptogenic cortex undergoing fibrillary gliosis after a local injury. *Brain Res.* 28:181-201.   128,130, 131

Grossman, R.G., Whiteside, L., and Hampton, T.L. (1969): The time course of evoked depolarization of cortical glial cells. *Brain Res.* 14:401-415.

Grundfest, H. (1966): Heterogeneity of excitable membrane: electrophysiological and pharmacological evidence and some consequences. *Ann. N.Y. Acad. Sci.* 137:901-949.   69

Gumnit, R.J. (1960): D.C. potential changes from auditory cortex of cat. *J. Neurophysiol.* 23:667-675.   127

Hafemann, D.R., Costin, A., and Tarby, T.J. (1969): Electrophysiological effects of enzymes introduced into the lateral geniculate body of the cat. *Exp. Neurol.* 27:238-247.   81

Hamberger, A. (1971): Amino acid uptake in neuronal and glial cell fractions from rabbit cerebral cortex. *Brain Res.* 31:169-178.

Harding, B.N. (1971): Dendro-dendritic synapses, including reciprocal synapses, in the ventrolateral nucleus of the monkey thalamus. *Brain Res.* 34:181-185.

Harris, E.J. (1972): *Transport and Accumulation in Biological Systems.* 3rd Ed. London: Butterworth, Inc. Baltimore: University Park Press.

Harris, W.F. and Scriven, L.E. (1971): Moving dislocations in cylindrical crystals cause waves of bending. I. Kink angle and wave types. *J. Mechanochem. Cell Motility* 1:33-40.

168

Page

Harth, E.M., Csermely, T.J., Beek, B., and Lindsay, R.D. (1970): Brain functions and neural dynamics. *J. Theor. Biol.* 26:93-120.

Hartman, H. and High, R. (1974): Bioconvection and morphogenesis in *Tetrahymena. J. Chem. Ecol.* (In press)   52,53

Hearon, J.Z. (1949a): The steady state kinetics of some biological systems: I. *Bull. Math. Biophys.* 11:29-50.   27

Hearon, J.Z. (1949b): The steady state kinetics of some biological systems: II. *Bull. Math. Biophys.* 11:83-95.   27

Hearon, J.Z. (1950a): Some cellular diffusion problems based on Onsager's generalization of Fick's Law. *Bull. Math. Biophys.* 12:135-159.   27

Hearon, J.Z. (1950b): The steady state kinetics of some biological systems: III. Thermodynamic aspects. *Bull. Math. Biophys.* 12:57-83.   27

Hearon, J.Z. (1950c): The steady state kinetics of some biological systems: IV. Thermodyanmic aspects. *Bull. Math. Biophys.* 12:85-106.   27

Hearon, J. (1953): The kinetics of linear systems with special reference to periodic reactions. *Bull. Math. Biophys.* 15:121-141.   60

Henn, F.A. and Hamberger, A. (1971): Glial cell function: uptake of transmitter substances. *Proc. Nat. Acad. Sci.* 68:2686-2690.

Henneman, E., Somjen, G., and Carpenter, D.O. (1965): Excitability and inhibitability of motoneurons of different sizes. *J. Neurophysiol.* 28:599-620.

Henneman, E., Somjen, G., and Carpenter, D.O. (1965): Functional significance of cell size in spinal motoneurons. *J. Neurophysiol.* 28:560-580.

Hern, J.E.C., Landgren, S., Phillips, C.G., and Porter, R. (1962): Selective excitation of corticofugal neurones by surface-anodal stimulation of the baboon's motor cortex. *J. Physiol.* 161:73-90.

Herschkowitz-Kaufman, M. (1970): Structures dissipatives dans une réaction chimique homogène. *C.R. Acad. Sci.* 270C:1049-1052.   31,32

Hess, B. and Boiteux, A. (1968): Control of glycolysis. *In: Regulatory Functions of Biological Membranes.* Järnefelt, J., ed. Amsterdam: Elsevier, pp. 148-162.   60,61

Higgins, J. (1964): A chemical mechanism for oscillation of glycolytic intermediates in yeast cells. *Proc. Nat. Acad. Sci.* 51:989-994.   61,62

Hill, T.L. (1967): Electric fields and the cooperativity of biological membranes. *Proc. Nat. Acad. Sci.* 58:111-114.   53

Hill, T.L. and Kedem, O. (1967): Studies in irreversible dynamics. 3. Models for steady state and active transport across membranes. *J. Theor. Biol.* 10:399-441.   66

Hilmy, M. and Somjen, G. (1968): Distribution and tissue uptake of magnesium related to its pharmacological effects. *Am. J. Physiol.* 214:406-413.   84

Hirsch, H.V.B. and Spinelli, D.N. (1971): Modification of the distribution of receptive field orientation in cats by selective visual exposure during development. *Exp. Brain Res.* 13:509-527.

Hodgkin, A.L. (1964): *The Conduction of the Nervous Impulse.* Springfield, Ill.: C.C Thomas.   57

Hodgkin, A.L. and Huxley, A.F. (1952): A quantitative description of membrane current and its application to conduction and excitation in nerve. *J. Physiol.* 117:500-544.   27,29, 67

Hodgkin, A.L. and Katz, B. (1949): The effect of sodium ions on the electrical activity of the giant axon of the squid. *J. Physiol.* 108:37-77.   27

Horowitz, J.M. (1972): Evoked activity of single units and neural populations in the hippocampus of the cat. *Electroencephalogr. Clin. Neurophysiol.* 32: 227-240.

Horowitz, J.M. and Freeman, W.J. (1972): Evoked activity of single units and neural populations in the hippocampus of the cat. *Electroencephalogr. Clin. Neurophysiol.* 32:227-240.

Householder, A.S. and Landahl, H.D. (1945): *Mathematical Biophysics of the Central Nervous System.* Bloomington, Ind.: Principia Press.   30

Hubel, D.H. and Wiesel, T.N. (1970): The period of susceptibility to the physiological effects of unilateral eye closure in kittens. *J. Physiol.* 206:419-436.

Hull, C.L. (1952): *A Behavior System.* New Haven: Yale University Press.   111

Humphrey, D.R. (1968a): Re-analysis of the antidromic cortical response. I. Potentials evoked by stimulation of the isolated pyramidal tract. *Electroencephalogr. Clin. Neurophysiol.* 24:116-129.

Humphrey, D.R. (1968b): Re-analysis of the antidromic cortical response. II. On the contribution of cell discharge and PSPs to the evoked potentials. *Electroencephalogr. Clin. Neurophysiol.* 25:421-442.

Huxley, J.S. and De Beer, G.R. (1934): *Elements of Experimental Embryology.* Cambridge: Cambridge University Press, pp. 133-192; 1963 Ed., New York: Hafner Press.   65

Jensen, D. (1966): The hagfish. *Sci. Am.* 214:82-90.

Jöbsis, F.F., O'Connor, M., Vitale, A., and Vreman, H. (1971): Intracellular redox changes in functioning cerebral cortex. I. Metabolic effects of epileptiform activity. *J. Neurophysiol.* 34:735-749.   124

John, E.R. (1972): Switchboard versus statistical theories of learning and memory. *Science* 177:850-864.   94,98

Josephson, R.K., Reiss, R.F., and Worthy, R.M. (1961): A simulation study of a diffuse conducting system based on coelenterate nerve nets. *J. Theor. Biol.* 1:460-487. 73

Joyner, R. and Somjen, G. (1972): A model simulating the contribution of glia to sustained potential shifts of central nervous tissue. *In: 26th Annual Meeting of the American EEG Society. (Abstr. 3)* 129

Kaczmarek, L.K. and Adey, W.R. (1973): The efflux of $^{45}Ca^{2+}$ and $[^3H]\gamma$-amino-butyric acid from cat cerebral cortex. *Brain Res.* 63:331-342. 81,82

Kaczmarek, L.K. and Adey, W.R. (1974a): Some chemical and electrophysiological effects of glutamate in cerebral cortex. *J. Neurobiol.* (In press) 84

Kaczmarek, L.K. and Adey, W.R. (1974b): Weak electric gradients change ionic and transmitter fluxes in cortex. *Brain Res.* 66:537-540. 84,85

Kaissling, K.-E. (1971): Insect olfaction. *In: Handbook of Sensory Physiology, Vol. IV. Chemical Senses, Part 1.* Beidler, L.M., ed. New York: Springer-Verlag, pp. 382-386. 144

Kandel, E.R. and Spencer, W.A. (1961): Electrophysiology of hippocampal neurons. II. After-potentials and repetitive firing. *J. Neurophysiol.* 24:243-259.

Kandel, E.R. and Spencer, W.A. (1961): Excitation and inhibition of single pyramidal cells during hippocampal seizure. *Exp. Neurol.* 4:162-179.

Kandel, E.R., Spencer, W.A., and Brinley, F.J., Jr. (1961): Electrophysiology of hippocampal neurons. I. Sequential invasion and synaptic organization. *J. Neurophysiol.* 24:225-242. 107

Karahashi, Y. and Goldring, S. (1966): Intracellular potentials from "idle" cells in cerebral cortex of cat. *Electroencephalogr. Clin. Neurophysiol.* 20:600-607.

Katchalsky, A. (1963): Nonequilibrium thermodynamics. *Int. Sci. Tech.* 22:43-49, 117-119. Also *In: Modern Science and Technology.* Colburn, R., et al., eds. New York: D. Van Nostrand, 1965, pp. 194-201.

Katchalsky, A. (1971): Biological flow structures and their relation to chemico-diffusional coupling. *In: Carriers and Specificity in Membranes.* Eigen, M. and De Maeyer, L. *Neurosciences Res. Prog. Bull.* 9:397-413. Also *In: Neurosciences Research Symposium Summaries, Vol. 6.* Schmitt, F.O. et al., eds. Cambridge, Mass.: M.I.T. Press, 1972, pp. 397-413. 42,46

Katchalsky, A. and Curran, P.F. (1965): *Nonequilibrium Thermodynamics in Biophysics.* Cambridge, Mass.: Harvard University Press.

Katchalsky, A. and Oster, G. (1969): Chemico-diffusional coupling in biomembranes. *In: The Molecular Basis of Membrane Function.* Tosteson, D.C., ed. Englewood Cliffs, N.J.: Prentice-Hall, Inc., pp. 1-44.

Katchalsky, A. and Spangler, R. (1968): Dynamics of membrane processes. *Q. Rev. Biophys.* 1:127-175. 65

Katz, B. and Schmitt, O.H. (1940): Electric interaction between two adjacent nerve fibres. *J. Physiol.* 97:471-488.

Katz, B. and Schmitt, O.H. (1942): A note on interaction between nerve fibres.   138
J. Physiol. 100:369-371.

Kauffman, S. (1972): Limit-cycle oscillations. *In: Genesis of Neuronal Patterns.*   59
Edds, M.E., Barkley, D.S., and Fambrough, D.M. *Neurosciences Res. Prog. Bull.*
10:319-325.

Kauffman, S. (1974): Phase dependent lobopodial contact paralysis. *Exp. Cell Res.*   59
(In press)

Kauffman, S. and Wille, J.J. (1974): The control of mitosis in *Physarum*   60
polycephalum by a continuous biochemical oscillator. *Exp. Cell Res.* (In press)

Kawamura, H. and Sawyer, C.H. (1965): Elevation in brain temperature during   63
paradoxical sleep. *Science* 150:912-913.

Kawamura, H., Whitmoyer, D.I., and Sawyer, C.H. (1966): Temperature changes in   63
the rabbit brain during paradoxical sleep. *Electroencephalogr. Clin. Neuro-*
physiol. 21:469-477.

Keizer, J. and Fox, R.F. (1974): Qualms regarding the range of validity of the   42
Glansdorff-Prigogine criterion for stability of non-equilibrium states. *Proc. Nat.*
Acad. Sci. 71:192-196.

Keller, E.F. and Segel, L.A. (1970): Initiation of slime mold aggregation viewed as   49,51
an instability. *J. Theor. Biol.* 26:399-415.

Kelly, J., Krnjević, K., and Somjen, G. (1969): Divalent cations and electrical
properties of cortical cells. *J. Neurobiol.* 1:197-208.

Kemény, A., Boldizsár, H., and Pethes, G. (1961): The distribution of cations in   84
plasma and cerebrospinal fluid following infusion of solutions of salts of sodium,
potassium, magnesium and calcium. *J. Neurochem.* 7:218-227.

Kerner, E.H. (1971): Statistical-mechanical theories in biology. *Adv. Chem. Phys.*   56
19:325-352.

Knight, B.W. (1972): Dynamics of encoding in a population of neurons. *J. Gen.*   104
Physiol. 59:734-766.

Köhler, W., Neff, W.D., and Wegener, J. (1955): Currents of the auditory cortex in
the cat. *J. Cell. Comp. Physiol.* 45(Suppl. 1):1-24.

Köhler, W. and O'Connell, D.N. (1957): Currents of the visual cortex of the cat.
J. Cell. Comp. Physiol. 49:(Suppl. 2):1-43.

Konorski, J. (1966): The nature of anodal current effects. *In: Brain Mechanisms in*
Conditioning and Learning. Livingston, R.B. *Neurosciences Res. Prog. Bull.*
4:298-299. Also *In: Neurosciences Research Symposium Summaries, Vol. 2.*
Schmitt, F.O. et al., eds. Cambridge, Mass.: M.I.T. Press, 1967, pp. 153-154.

Page

Kopell, N. and Howard, L.N. (1973): Horizontal bands in the Belousov reaction. 33,34
Science 180:1171-1173.

Korn, H. and Bennett, M.V.L. (1971): Dendritic and somatic impulse initiation in 92
fish oculomotor neurons during vestibular nystagmus. *Brain Res.* 27:169-175.

Korn, H. and Bennett, M.V.L. (1972): Electrotonic coupling between teleost 93
oculomotor neurons; restriction to somatic regions and function of somatic and
dendritic sites of impulse initiation. *Brain Res.* 38:433-439.

Koschmieder, E.L. (1966): On convection on a uniformly heated plane. *Beitr.* 14
Physik Atmos. 39:1-11.

Koshland, D.E., Jr. (1963): The role of flexibility in enzyme action. *Cold Spring* 65
Harbor Symp. Quant. Biol. 28:473-482.

Kraft, M.S., Obrist, W.D., and Pribram, K.H. (1960): The effect of irritative lesions
of the striate cortex on learning of visual discriminations in monkeys. *J. Comp.*
Physiol. Psychol. 53:17-22.

Krampitz, G. and Fox, S.W. (1969): The condensation of the adenylates of the
amino acids common to protein. *Proc. Nat. Acad. Sci.* 62:399-406.

Kriebel, M.E., Bennett, M.V.L., Waxman, S.G., and Pappas, G.D. (1969): 93
Oculomotor neurons in fish: electrotonic coupling and multiple sites of 'impulse'
initiation. *Science* 166:520-524.

Kuffler, S.W. (1967): Neuroglial cells: physiological properties and a postassium
mediated effect of neuronal activity on the glial membrane potential. *Proc. Roy.*
Soc. B 168:1-21.

Kuffler, S.W. and Nicholls, J.G. (1966): The physiology of neuroglial cells. *Ergeb.*
Physiol. 57:1-90.

Kuffler, S.W., Nicholls, J.G., and Orkand, R.K. (1966): Physiological properties of 85,130
glial cells in the central nervous system of amphibia. *J. Neurophysiol.*
29:768-787.

Kuhn, Th.S. (1970): *The Structure of Scientific Revolutions.* 2nd Ed. Chicago: 11
University of Chicago Press.

Kupfermann, I. (1965): Effects of cortical polarization on visual discriminations.
Exp. Neurol. 12:179-189.

Landau, W.M., Bishop, G.H., and Clare, M.H. (1964): Analysis of the form and
distribution of evoked cortical potentials under the influence of polarizing
currents. *J. Neurophysiol.* 27:788-813.

Lange, O.R. (1965): *Wholes and Parts: A General Theory of System Behaviour.* 95,96
New York: Pergamon Press.

Lebovitz, R.B., Dichter, M., and Spencer, W.A. (1971): Recurrent excitation in the 107
CA3 region of cat hippocampus. *Int. J. Neurosci.* 2:99-108.

Page

Lefelhocz, J.F. (1972): The color blind traffic light: an undergraduate kinetics experiment using an oscillating reaction. *J. Chem. Educ.* 49:312-314.   32,34

Lefever, R. (1968): Dissipative structures in chemical systems. *J. Chem. Phys.* 49:4977-4978.   41,42

Lefever, R. and Nicolis, G. (1971): Chemical instabilities and sustained oscillations. *J. Theor. Biol.* 30:267-284.   40

Libet, B. and Gerard, R.W. (1941): Steady potential fields and neurone activity. *J. Neurophysiol.* 4:438-455.

Lickey, M. (1969): Autorhythmic activity in single neurons. *In: Slow Electrical Phenomena in the Central Nervous System.* Adey, W.R. *Neurosciences Res. Prog. Bull.* 7:121-127. Also *In: Neurosciences Research Symposium Summaries, Vol. 4.* Schmitt, F.O. et al., eds. Cambridge, Mass.: M.I.T. Press, 1970, pp. 47-53.   71

Liesegang, R.E. (1906): Geschichtete Structuren. *Z. Anorg. Chem.* 48:364-366.   30

Lodin, S., Hartman, J., Kage, M.P., Korinková, P., and Booher, J. (1971): Potassium-induced hydration in cultured neural tissue. *Neurobiology* 1:69-85.   150

Loefer, J.B. and Mefferd, R.B., Jr. (1952): Concerning pattern formation by free-swimming microorganisms. *Am. Natural.* 86:325-329.

Loewenstein, W.R. (1968a): Communication through cell junctions. Implications in growth and differentiation. *In: The Emergence of Order in Developing Systems.* Locke, M., ed. New York: Academic Press, pp. 151-183.   64,70

Loewenstein, W.R. (1968b): Some reflections on growth and differentiation. *Perspect. Biol. Med.* 11:260-272.

Lotka, A.J. (1920): Undamped oscillations derived from the law of mass action. *J. Am. Chem. Soc.* 42:1595-1599.   22

Lotka, A.J. (1924): *Elements of Physical Biology.* Baltimore: Williams and Wilkins.   22

Lotka, A.J. (1956): *Elements of Mathematical Biology.* 2nd Ed. New York: Dover Publications.   22

Lux, H.D. and Pollen, D.A. (1966): Electrical constants of neurons in the motor cortex of the cat. *J. Neurophysiol.* 29:207-220.

Luzzati, V. and Husson F. (1962): The structure of the liquid-crystalline phases of lipid-water systems. *J. Cell Biol.* 12:207-219.   18

McCulloch, W.S. and Pitts, W. (1943): A logical calculus of the ideas immanent in nervous activity. *Bull. Math. Biophys.* 5:115-133.   73

MacKay, D.M. (1957): The stabilization of perception during voluntary activity. *In: Proceedings of the XV International Congress of Psychology.* Amsterdam: North-Holland Publishing Co., pp. 284-285.

MacKay, D.M. (1962): Theoretical models of space perception. *In: Aspects of the Theory of Artificial Intelligence.* Muses, C.A., ed. New York: Plenum Press, pp. 83-104.

MacKay, D.M. (1966): Cerebral organization and the conscious control of action. *In: Brain and Conscious Experience.* Eccles, J.C., ed. Berlin-Heidelberg-New York: Springer-Verlag, pp. 422-445.

MacKay, D.M. (1970): Mislocation of test flashes during saccadic image displacements. *Nature* 227:731-733.

MacKay, D.M. (1972): Visual stability. *Invest. Ophthalmol.* 11:518-524.

MacKay, D.M. (1972): Voluntary eye movements as questions. *In: Cerebral Control of Eye Movements and Motion Perception.* Dichgans, J. and Bizzi, E., eds. Basel: S. Karger, pp. 369-376.

MacKay, D.M. (1973): Visual stability and voluntary eye movements. *In: Handbook of Sensory Physiology, Vol. VII/3A. Visual Centers in the Brain.* Jung, R., ed. New York: Springer-Verlag, pp. 307-331.

Malhotra, S.K. and Van Harreveld, A. (1966): Distribution of extracellular material in central white matter. *J. Anat.* 100:99-110.

Malhotra, S.K. and Van Harreveld, A. (1968): Molecular organization of the membranes of cells and cellular organelles. *In: Biological Basis of Medicine, Vol. 1.* Bittar, E.E. and Bittar, N., eds. London: Academic Press, pp. 3-68.

Martins-Ferreira, H. and de Oliveira Castro, G. (1966): Light-scattering changes accompanying spreading depression in isolated retina. *J. Neurophysiol.* 29:715-726.

May, R.M. (1972): Limit cycles in predator-prey communities. *Science* 177:900-902.

Melzack, R. and Casey, K.L. (1967): Localized temperature changes evoked in the brain by somatic stimulation. *Exp. Neurol.* 17:276-292.

Meszler, R.M., Pappas, G.S., and Bennett, M.V.L. (1972): Morphological demonstration of electrotonic coupling by way of presynaptic fibers. *Brain Res.* 36:412-415.

Mollica, A. and Rossi, G.F. (1954): Attivita de singule unita del systema pyramidale durante la polarizzazione della zona corticale motrice. *Arch. Fiziol.* 54:219-230.

Monod, J., Changeux, J.-P., and Jacob, F. (1963): Allosteric proteins and cellular control systems. *J. Mol. Biol.* 6:306-329.

Morrell, F. (1956): Interseizure disturbances in focal epilepsy. *Neurology* 6:327-334.

Morrell, F. (1957): An anatomical and physiological analysis of electrocortical conditioning. *In: Proceedings of the First International Congress on Neurosciences, Brussels,* pp. 377-391.

Morrell, F. (1957): Effect of experimental epilepsy on conditioned electrical potentials. *Univ. Minn. Med. Bull.* 29:82-102.

Morrell, F. (1957): Effets de lésions épileptiques focales sur la formation de connexions temporaires chez le singe. *In: Conditionnement et Réactivité en electroencéphalographie. Electroencephalogr. Clin. Neurophysiol.* 6(Suppl.): 51-74.

Morrell, F. (1960): Microelectrode and steady potential studies suggesting a dendritic locus of closure. *In: The Moscow Colloquium of Electroencephalography of Higher Nervous Activity.* Jasper, H.H. and Smirnov, G.D., eds. *Electroencephalogr. Clin. Neurophysiol.* 13(Suppl.):65-79.

Morrell, F. (1961a): Effect of anodal polarization on the firing pattern of single cortical cells. *Ann. N.Y. Acad. Sci.* 92:860-876.   135,137

Morrell, F. (1961b): Electrophysiological contributions to the neural basis of learning. *Physiol. Rev.* 41:443-494.

Morrell, F. (1963): Information storage in nerve cells. *In: Information Storage and Neural Control.* Fields, W.S. and Abbott, W., eds. Springfield, Ill.: C.C Thomas, pp. 189-229.

Morrell, F. (1966): Central events during conditioning. *In: Brain Mechanisms in   137 Conditioning and Learning.* Livingston, R.B. *Neurosciences Res. Prog. Bull.* 4:292-298, 301-303. Also *In: Neurosciences Research Symposium Summaries, Vol. 2.* Schmitt, F.O. et al., eds. Cambridge, Mass.: M.I.T. Press, 1967, pp. 149-152, 154-159.

Morrell, F. (1967): Electrical signs of sensory coding. *In: The Neurosciences: A Study Program.* Quarton, G.C., Melnechuk, T., and Schmitt, F.O., eds. New York: Rockefeller University Press, pp. 452-469.

Morrell, F. (1969): Neuronal and behavioral conditioned responses with imposed DC gradients. *In: Slow Electrical Phenomena in the Central Nervous System.* Adey, W.R. *Neurosciences Res. Prog. Bull.* 7:92-97. Also *In: Neurosciences Research Symposium Summaries, Vol. 4.* Schmitt, F.O. et al., eds. Cambridge, Mass.: M.I.T. Press, 1970, pp. 18-23.

Morrell, F. and Jasper, H.H. (1956): Electrographic studies of the formation of temporary connections in the brain. *Electroencephalogr. Clin. Neurophysiol.* 8:201-215.

Morrell, F. and Naitoh, P. (1962): Effect of cortical polarization on a conditioned   137 avoidance response. *Exp. Neurol.* 6:507-523.

Morrell, F., Roberts, L., and Jasper, H.H. (1956): Effect of focal epileptogenic lesions and their ablation upon conditioned electrical responses of the brain in the monkey. *Electroencephalogr. Clin. Neurophysiol.* 8:217-236.

Movshon, J.A., Chambers, B.E.I., and Blakemore, C. (1972): Interocular transfer in normal humans, and those who lack stereopsis. *Perception* 1:483-490.

Page

Nashold, B., Somjen, G., and Friedman, H. (1972): Paresthesias and EEG potentials evoked by stimulation of the dorsal funiculi in man. *Exp. Neurol.* 36:273-287.

Nelson, P.G. (1966): Interaction between spinal motoneurons of the cat. *J. Neurophysiol.* 29:275-287.   137

Nelson, P.G. and Frank, K. (1964): Extracellular potential fields of single spinal motoneurons. *J. Neurophysiol.* 27:913-927.   137

Nicholson, C. (1971): Mathematical model of field potentials in a cerebellar cortex and other laminar neural tissues. *Biophysical Society Abstracts.* Fifteenth Annual Meeting, New Orleans, La. 11:244a.

Nicholson, C. and Llinás, R. (1971): Field potentials in the alligator cerebellum and theory of their relationship to Purkinje cell dendritic spikes. *J. Neurophysiol.* 34:509-531.

Norton, S. and Jewett, E.J. (1965): Frequencies of slow potential oscillations in cortex of cats. *Electroencephalogr. Clin. Neurophysiol.* 19:377-386.   63

O'Leary, J.L. and Goldring, S. (1964): D-C potentials of the brain. *Physiol. Rev.* 44:91-125.

Omura, Y., Lee, K., and Jeronimo, M. (1972): Stimulation (stim.) of excitable cell membranes by capacitative current (Ic) and rapidly-changing electro-magnetic field (R-C-EMF) without direct contact between electrodes and the cell. *Fed. Proc.* 31:298. (Abstr.)

Oppelt, W.W., Owens, E.S., and Rall, D.P. (1963): Calcium exchange between blood and cerebrospinal fluid. *Life Sci.* 8:599-605.   84

Oster, G.F. and Desoer, C.A. (1971): Tellegen's theorem and thermodynamic inequalities. *J. Theor. Biol.* 32:219-241.

Oster, G., Perelson, A., and Katchalsky, A. (1971): Network thermodynamics. *Nature* 234:393-399.

Othmer, H.G. (1971): Interactions of reaction and diffusion in open systems. Ph.D. Dissertation, University of Minnesota, Minneapolis, Minnesota.

Othmer, H.G. and Scriven, L.E. (1969): Interactions of reaction and diffusion in open systems. *Ind. Eng. Chem.* 8:302-313.

Othmer, H.G. and Scriven, L.E. (1971): Instability and dynamic pattern in cellular networks. *J. Theor. Biol.* 32:507-537.   38,58, 127

Othmer, H.G. and Scriven, L.E. (1974): Non-linear aspects of dynamic pattern in cellular networks. *J. Theor. Biol.* 43:83-112.   58

Paecht-Horowitz, M., Berger, J., and Katchalsky, A. (1970): Prebiotic synthesis of polypeptides by heterogeneous condensation of amino-acid adenylates. *Nature* 228:636-639.   45

Pantin, C.F.A. (1952): The elementary nervous system. *Proc. Roy. Soc. B* 140:147-168.

73

Pappas, G.D., Asada, Y., and Bennett, M.V.L. (1971): Morphological correlates of increased coupling resistance at an electrotonic synapse. *J. Cell Biol.* 49: 173-188.

90,91

Payton, B.W., Bennett, M.V.L., and Pappas, G.D. (1969): Permeability and structure of junctional membranes at an electrotonic synapse. *Science* 166:1641-1643.

90,91

Perkel, D.H. and Bullock, T.H. (1968): *Neural Coding. Neurosciences Res. Prog. Bull.* 6:221-348. Also *In: Neurosciences Research Symposium Summaries, Vol. 3.* Schmitt, F.O. et al., eds. Cambridge, Mass.: M.I.T. Press, 1969, pp. 405-527.

109

Peronnet, F., Anninos, P.A., and Elul, R. (1971): Mapping of nerve cell populations with disc-type EEG electrodes. *In: First European Biophysics Congress, 14-17 September, 1971, Baden.* Broda, E., Locker, A., and Springer-Lederer, H., eds. Vienna: Verlag der Wiener Medizinischen Akademie, pp. 231-235.

Pettigrew, J., Olson, C., and Barlow, H.B. (1973): Kitten visual cortex: short-term, stimulus-induced changes in connectivity. *Science* 180:1202-1203.

Pittendrigh, C.S. (1974): Circadian oscillations in cells and the circadian organization of multicellular systems. *In: The Neurosciences: Third Study Program.* Schmitt, F.O. and Worden, F.G., eds. Cambridge, Mass.: M.I.T. Press, pp. 437-458.

71

Pitts, W. and McCulloch, W.S. (1947): How we know universals: the perception of auditory and visual forms. *Bull. Math. Biophys.* 9:127-147.

98

Platt, J. (1970): Hierarchical growth. *Bull. Atom. Sci.* 26:2-48.

11,20

Poggio, G.F. and Viernstein, L.J. (1964): Time series analysis of impulse sequences of thalamic somatic sensory neurons. *J. Neurophysiol.* 27:517-545.

76

Pollen, D.A. (1964): Intracellular studies of cortical neurons during thalamic induced wave and spike. *Electroencephalogr. Clin. Neurophysiol.* 17:398-404.

Pollen, D.A. (1969): Discussion: On the generation of neocortical potentials. *In: Basic Mechanisms of the Epilepsies.* Jasper, H.H., Ward, A.A., Jr., and Pope, A., eds. Boston: Little, Brown and Co., pp. 411-420.

Pollen, D.A., Lee, J.R., and Taylor, J.H. (1971): How does the striate cortex begin the reconstruction of the visual world? *Science* 173:74-77.

Pollen, D.A. and Richardson, E.P., Jr. (1972): Intracellular microelectrode studies at the border zone of glial scars developing after penetrating wounds and freezing lesions of the sensorimotor area of the cat. *Recent Contributions to Neurophysiology. EEG Supplement No. 31* Cordeau, J.P. and Gloor, P., eds. Amsterdam: Elsevier, pp. 27-41.

Pollen, D.A. and Sie, P.-G. (1964): Analysis of thalamic induced wave and spike by modifications in cortical excitability. *Electroencephalogr. Clin. Neurophysiol.* 17:154-163.

Ponnamperuma, C., Sagan, C., and Mariner, R. (1963): Synthesis of adenosine triphosphate under possible primitive earth conditions. *Nature* 199:222-226.

Porter, R., Adey, W.R., and Kado, R.T. (1964): Measurement of electrical impedance in the human brain. *Neurology* 14:1002-1012.   81

Prigogine, I. (1969): Structure, dissipation and life. *In: Theoretical Physics and Biology.* Marois, M., ed. Amsterdam: North-Holland Publishing Co., pp. 23-52.   31,65

Prigogine, I., Lefever, R., Goldbetter, A., and Herschkowitz-Kaufman, M. (1969): Symmetry breaking instabilities in biological systems. *Nature* 223:913-916.   31

Prigogine, I. and Nicolis, G. (1971): Biological order, structure and instabilities. *Q. Rev. Biophys.* 4:107-148.

Prince, D.A., Lux, H.D., and Neher, E. (1973): Measurement of extracellular potassium activity in cat cortex. *Brain Res.* 50:489-495.   148

Proctor, F., Pinto-Hamacy, T., and Kupfermann, I. (1964): Cortical stimulation during learning in rabbits. *Neuropsychologia* 2:305-310.

Purpura, D.P. (1959): Nature of electrocortical potentials and synaptic organizations in cerebral and cerebellar cortex. *Int. Rev. Neurobiol.* 1:47-163.

Purpura, D.P. (1967): Comparative physiology of dendrites. *In: The Neurosciences: A Study Program.* Quarton, G.C., Melnechuk, T., and Schmitt, F.O., eds. New York: Rockefeller University Press, pp. 372-393.

Purpura, D.P. (1968): Excitability changes in dendrites of thalamic neurons during prolonged activation. *Brain Res.* 10:457-459.

Purpura, D.P. (1971): Dendrites: heterogeneity in form and function. *Handb. Electroencephalogr. Clin. Neurophysiol.* 1:1B-3-1B-17.

Purpura, D.P. (1971): Synaptogenesis in mammalian cortex: problems and perspectives. *In: Brain Development and Behavior.* Sterman, M.B., McGinty, D.J., and Adinolfi, A.M., eds. New York: Academic Press, pp. 23-41.

Purpura, D.P. (1972): Ontogenetic models in studies of cortical seizure activities. *In: Models of Experimental Epilepsy.* Purpura, D., et al., eds. New York: Raven Press, pp. 532-536.

Purpura, D.P., Desiraju, T., Prelevic, S., and Santini, M. (1968): Excitability changes in dendrites of thalamic neurons during prolonged synaptic activation. *Brain Res.* 10:457-459.

Purpura, D.P. and McMurtry, J.G. (1965): Intracellular activities and evoked potential changes during polarization of motor cortex. *J. Neurophysiol.* 28:166-185.   133,139

Purpura, D.P. and Shofer, R.J. (1972): Excitatory action of dibutyryl cyclic adenosine monophosphate on immature cerebral cortex. *Brain Res.* 38:179-181.

Rall, W. (1962): Electrophysiology of a dendritic neuron model. *Biophys. J.* 2:145-167.

Rall, W. (1962): Theory of physiological properties of dendrites. *Ann. N.Y. Acad. Sci.* 96:1071-1092.

Rall, W. (1964): Theoretical significance of dendritic trees for neuronal input-output relations. *In: Neural Theory and Modeling.* Reiss, R.F., ed. Stanford: Stanford University Press, pp. 73-97.

Rall, W. (1967): Distinguishing theoretical synaptic potentials computed for different soma-dendritic distributions of synaptic input. *J. Neurophysiol.* 30:1072-1193.

Rall, W. (1969): Distributions of potentials in cylindrical coordinates and time constants for a membrane cylinder. *Biophys. J.* 9:1509-1541.

Rall, W. (1969): Time constants and electrotonic length of membrane cylinders and neurons. *Biophys. J.* 9:1483-1508.

Rall, W. (1970a): Cable properties of dendrites and effect of synaptic location. *In: Excitatory Synaptic Mechanisms.* Andersen, P. and Jansen, J.K.S., eds. Oslo: Universitetsforlaget, pp. 175-187.   90

Rall, W. (1970b): Dendritic neuron theory and dendrodendritic synapses in a simple cortical system. *In: The Neurosciences: Second Study Program.* Schmitt, F.O., editor-in-chief. New York: Rockefeller University Press, pp. 552-565.

Rall, W. and Shepherd, G.M. (1968): Theoretical reconstruction of field potentials   28,105
and dendrodendritic synaptic interactions in olfactory bulb. *J. Neurophysiol.* 31:884-915.

Ramón y Cajal, S. (1955): *Histologie du Système Nerveux de L'Homme et des*   130,131
Vertébrés, Vol. II. Madrid: Consejo Superior de Investigaciones Cientificas, Instituto Ramón y Cajal, p. 586.

Ransom, B.R. and Goldring, S. (1973): Slow hyperpolarization in cells presumed to   121
be glia in cerebral cortex of cat. *J. Neurophysiol.* 36:879-892.

Rashevsky, N. (1933): Outline of a physico-mathematical theory of excitation and inhibition. *Protoplasma* 20:42-56.

Rashevsky, N. (1938): *Mathematical Biophysics.* Chicago: University of Chicago   25,30
Press; 2nd Ed., Chicago: University of Chicago Press, 1948; 3rd Ed., New York: Dover Publications, 1960.

Rayleigh, Lord (1916): On convective currents in a horizontal layer of fluid, when   13
the higher temperature is on the under side. *Philos. Mag.* 32:529-546.

Raymond, S.A. and Lettvin, J.Y. (1969): Influences on axonal conduction. *Q. Prog. Rep. M.I.T. Res. Lab. Electr.* 92:431-435.

Rebert, C.S. (1969): DC and multiple-unit recording in lateral geniculate body of the cat. *In: Proceedings of the 77th Annual American Psychological Association, 1969.* 4:215-216.

Rebert, C.S. (1973): A technique for simultaneous measurement of DC and multiple unit responses. *Electroencephalogr. Clin. Neurophysiol.* 34:326-328.

Reiss, R.F., ed. (1964): *Neural Theory and Modeling.* Stanford: Stanford University Press.

Revel, J.P. and Karnovsky, M.J. (1967): Hexagonal array of subunits in intercellular junctions of the mouse heart and liver. *J. Cell Biol.* 33:C7-C12.

Revel, J.P., Yee, A.G., and Hudspeth, A.J. (1971): Gap junctions between electrotonically coupled cells in tissue culture and in brown fat. *Proc. Nat. Acad. Sci.* 68:2924-2927.

Robbins, W.J. (1952): Patterns formed by motile *Euglena gracilis* var. *bacillaris. Bull. Torrey Bot. Club.* 79:107-109.

Robertson, A. and Cohen, M.H. (1972): Control of developing fields. *Annu. Rev. Biophys. Bioeng.* 1:409-464.

Rosen, R. (1970): *Dynamical Systems Theory in Biology: Stability Theory and Its Application. Vol. 1.* New York: Wiley-Interscience.

Rosenthal, M. and Somjen G. (1971): Sustained evoked potentials, spreading depression and metabolic activity of the cerebral cortex measured in situ. *Proc. Int. Union Physiol. Sci.* 9:479.

Rosenthal, M. and Somjen, G. (1973): Spreading depression, sustained potential shifts, and metabolic activity of cerebral cortex of cats. *J. Neurophysiol.* 36:739-749.

Rowland, V. (1967): Steady potential phenomena of cortex. *In: The Neurosciences: A Study Program.* Quarton, G.C., Melnechuk, T., and Schmitt, F.O., eds. New York: Rockefeller University Press, pp. 482-495.

Rowland, V. (1968): Cortical steady potential (direct current potential) in reinforcement and learning. *In: Progress in Physiological Psychology, Vol. 2.* Stellar, E. and Sprague, J.M., eds. New York: Academic Press, pp. 1-77.

Rowland, V. and Anderson, R. (1971): Brain steady potential shifts. *In: Progress in Physiological Psychology, Vol. 4.* Stellar, E. and Sprague, J.M., eds. New York: Academic Press, pp. 37-51.

Rowland, V. and Dines, G. (1973): Cortical steady potential shift in relation to the rhythmic electrocorticogram and multiple unit activity. *In: Bioelectric Recording Techniques. Part A, Cellular Processes and Brain Potentials.* Thompson, R.F. and Patterson, M.M., eds. New York: Academic Press, pp. 369-385.

Page

Rusinov, V.S. (1953): An electrophysiological analysis of the connecting function   137
in the cerebral cortex in the presence of a dominant region area. *In: Proceedings of the XIX International Congress on Physiology, Montreal.* (Abstr.)

Ruspini, E.H. (1969): A new approach to clustering. *Inform. Control* 15:22-32.

Ruspini, E.H. (1970): Numerical methods for fuzzy clustering. *Inform. Sci.* 2:319-350.

Russell, I.S. and Ochs, S. (1961): One-trial interhemispheric transfer of a learning engram. *Science* 133:1077-1078.

Sastre, A. (1972): Cooperative interactions between endogenously active cells.   72
Session in Biomathematics, AAAS Meeting, December, 1972. (Abstr.)

Sayers, G. and Beall, R.J. (1973): Isolated adrenal cortex cells: hypersensitivity to   144
adrenocorticotropic hormone after hypophysectomy. *Science* 179:1330-1331.

Schmitt, F.O. (1969): Brain cell membranes and their microenvironment. *In: Brain Cell Microenvironment.* Schmitt, F.O. and Samson, F.E. *Neurosciences Res. Prog. Bull.* 7:281-300. Also *In: Neurosciences Research Symposium Summaries, Vol. 4.* Schmitt, F.O. et al., eds. Cambridge, Mass.: M.I.T. Press, 1970, pp. 195-214.

Schmitt, F.O. and Samson, F.E. (1969): *Brain cell microenvironment. Neuro-*   58,80,
sciences Res. Prog. Bull. 7:275-417. Also *In: Neurosciences Research Sympo-*   81
sium Summaries, Vol. 4. Schmitt, F.O. et al., eds. Cambridge, Mass.: M.I.T. Press, 1970, pp. 191-325.

Schmitt, O.H. (1969): Biological information processing using the concept of interpenetrating domains. *In: Information Processing in the Nervous System.* Leibovic, K.N., ed. New York: Springer-Verlag, pp. 325-331.

Schmitt, O.H. (1972): Impedance and mutual impedance. *BioScience* 22:37-38.

Schulman, J.H. and Rideal, E.K. (1937): Molecular interaction in monolayers: 17
I. Complexes between large molecules. II. The action of haemolytic and agglutinating agents on lipo-protein monolayers. *Proc. Roy. Soc. B* 122:29-57.

Schwarz, G. (1970): Cooperative binding to linear biopolymers. 1. Fundamental   143
static and dynamic properties. *Eur. J. Biochem.* 12:442-453.

Sel'kov, E.E. (1968): Self-oscillations in glycolysis. 1. A simple kinetic model. *Eur. J. Biochem.* 4:79-86.

Shaffer, B.M. (1962): The acrasina. *Adv. Morphog.* 2:109-182.   50

Sheafor, P. and Rowland, V. (1973): Cortical steady potential shift and integrating   118
mass unit activity in forms of temporal conditioning. *Program and Abstracts, Society for Neuroscience.* Third Annual Meeting, San Diego, Calif., p. 117.

Sloper, J.J. (1971): Dendro-dendritic synapses in the primate motor cortex. *Brain*   86
Res. 34:186-192.

Page

Sloper, J.J. (1972): Gap junctions between dendrites in the primate neocortex.   86
Brain Res. 44:641-646.

Somjen, G.G. (1969): Sustained evoked potential changes of the spinal cord. *Brain*   121
Res. 12:268-272.

Somjen, G.G. (1970): Evoked sustained focal potentials and membrane potentials   121,122,
of neurons and of unresponsive cells of the spinal cord. *J. Neurophysiol.*   125
33:562-582.

Somjen, G.G. (1973): Electrogenesis of sustained potential shifts of the central   122,126,
nervous system. *Prog. Neurobiol.* 1:199-235.   129

Somjen, G., Carpenter, D.O., and Henneman, E. (1965): Responses of motoneurons
of different sizes to graded stimulation of supraspinal centers of the brain.
J. Neurophysiol. 28:958-965.

Spehlmann, R. and Kapp, H. (1964): Direct extracellular polarization of cortical
neurons with multibarreled microelectrodes. *Arch. Ital. Biol.* 102:74-93.

Spencer, H. (1880): *First Principles.* Reprinted from the 5th London Ed. New   11
York: A.L. Burt; 9th Ed., Philadelphia: David McKay.

Spencer, W.A. and Brookhart, J.M. (1966): Electrical patterns of augmenting and
recruiting waves in depths of sensorimotor cortex of cat. *J. Neurophysiol.*
24:26-49.

Spencer, W.A. and Brookhart, J.M. (1966): A study of spontaneous spindle waves
in sensorimotor cortex of cat. *J. Neurophysiol.* 24:50-65.

Spencer, W.A. and Kandel, E.R. (1961a): Electrophysiology of hippocampal   108
neurons. III. Firing level and time constant. *J. Neurophysiol.* 24:260-271.

Spencer, W.A. and Kandel, E.R. (1961b): Electrophysiology of hippocampal   139
neurons. IV. Fast prepotentials. *J. Neurophysiol.* 24:272-285.

Spencer, W.A. and Kandel, E.R. (1961c): Hippocampal neuron responses to   107,108,
selective activation of recurrent collaterals of hippocampofugal axons. *Exp.*   147
Neurol. 4:149-161.

Spiegelman, S. (1971): An approach to the experimental analysis of precellular   48
evolution. *Q. Rev. Biophys.* 4:213-253.

Spira, M.E. and Bennett, M.V.L. (1972a): Penicillin induced seizure activity in the
hatchet fish. *Brain Res.* 43:235-241.

Spira, M.E. and Bennett, M.V.L. (1972b): Synaptic control of electrotonic coupling   93
between neurons. *Brain Res.* 37:294-300.

Stamm, J.S. and Pribram, K.H. (1960): Effects of epileptogenic lesions in frontal
cortex on learning and retention in monkeys. *J. Neurophysiol.* 23:552-563.

Steinbach, A.B. and Bennett, M.V.L. (1971): Effects of divalent ions and drugs on synaptic transmission in phasic electroreceptors in a mormyrid fish. *J. Gen. Physiol.* 58:580-598.

Steinbach, A.B. and Bennett, M.V.L. (1971): Presynaptic actions of Ca and Mg and postsynaptic actions of glutamate at a sensory synapse. *Biol. Bull.* 141:403.

Steinman, G. (1967): Sequence generation in prebiological peptide synthesis. *Arch. Biochem. Biophys.* 119:76-82 and 121:533-539.

Steinman, G. and Cole, M. (1967): Synthesis of biologically pertinent peptides under possible primordial conditions. *Proc. Nat. Acad. Sci.* 58:735-742.

Stoeckenius, W. (1962): Some electron microscopical observations on liquid crystalline phases in lipid-water systems. *J. Cell Biol.* 12:221-229.   18

Strässler, S. and Kittel, C. (1965): Degeneracy and the order of the phase transformation in the molecular-field approximation. *Phys. Rev. (Series 2)* 139:A758-A760.   67

Strittmatter, W.J. and Somjen, G.G. (1973): Depression of sustained evoked potentials and glial depolarization in the spinal cord by barbiturates and by diphenylhydantoin. *Brain Res.* 55:333-342.   123,124

Strumwasser, F. (1965): The demonstration and manipulation of a circadian rhythm in a single neuron. *In: Circadian Clocks.* Aschoff, J., ed. Amsterdam: North-Holland Publishing Co., pp. 442-462.   71

Strumwasser, F. (1967): Tetrodotoxin reveals two stable states of the resting potential in a neuron generating endogenous bursts. *Physiologist* 10:318.   71

Strumwasser, F. (1968): Membrane and intracellular mechanism governing endogenous activity in neurons. *In: Physiological and Biochemical Aspects of Nervous Integration.* Carlson, F.D., ed. Englewood Cliffs, N.J.: Prentice-Hall, Inc., pp. 329-341.   60,71

Strumwasser, F. and Rosenthal, S. (1960): Prolonged and patterned direct extracellular stimulation of single neurons. *Am. J. Physiol.* 198:405-413.

Stryker, M. and Blakemore, C. (1972): Saccadic and disjunctive eye movements in cats. *Vision Res.* 12:2005-2013.

Tarby, T.J. and Adey, W.R. (1967): Cytological chemical identification of calcium in brain tissue. *Anat. Rec.* 157:331-332. (Abstr.)   85

Tasaki, I. (1968): *Nerve Excitation: A Macromolecular Approach.* Springfield, Ill.: C.C Thomas.   66

Teorell, T. (1959): Electrokinetic membrane process in relation to properties of excitable tissues. I. Experiments on oscillatory transport phenomena in artificial membranes. *J. Gen. Physiol.* 42:831-845.

Page

Teorell, T. (1959): Electrokinetic membrane process in relation to properties of excitable tissues. II. Some theoretical considerations. *J. Gen. Physiol.* 42: 847-863.

Teorell, T. (1962): Excitability phenomena in artificial membranes. *Biophys. J.* 2:27-52.

Terzuolo, C.A. and Bullock, T.H. (1956): Measurement of imposed voltage gradient   137
adequate to modulate neuronal firing. *Proc. Nat. Acad. Sci.* 42:687-694.

Trachtenberg, M.C. and Pollen, D.A. (1970): Neuroglia: biophysical properties and   128,129
physiologic function. *Science* 167:1248-1252.

Travis, R.P. and Clark, L.C., Jr. (1965): Changes in evoked brain oxygen sensory   63
stimulation and conditioning. *Electroencephalogr. Clin. Neurophysiol.* 19:
484-491.

Tsujiyama, Y. (1963): Normal and pathological figures of neuroglia stained with   130
Tsujiyama's methods. *In: Morphology of Neuroglia.* Nakai, J., ed. Springfield,
Ill.: C.C Thomas, pp. 165-179.

Tucker, L.E. and Pichon, Y. (1972): Electrical and radioisotope evidence for an
insect "blood-brain barrier." *Nature New Biol.* 236:126-127.

Turing, A.M. (1952): The chemical basis of morphogenesis. *Phil. Trans. Roy. Soc. B*   25,35.
237:37-72.   36.64

Ussing, H.H. and Zerahn, K. (1951): Active transport of sodium as the source of   127
electric current in the short-circuited isolated frog skin. *Acta Physiol. Scand.*
23:110-127.

Van der Loos, H. (1960): On dendro-dendritic junctions in the cerebral cortex. *In:*   86,87
Structure and Function of the Cerebral Cortex. Tower, D.B. and Schadé, J.P.,
eds. Amsterdam: Elsevier, pp. 36-42.

Van der Loos, H. (1963): Fine structure of synapses in the cerebral cortex. *Z.*   86
Zellforsch. Mikrosk. Anat. 60:815-825.

Van der Loos, H. (1964): Similarities and dissimilarities in submicroscopical   86
morphology of interneuronal contact sites of presumably different functional
character. *Prog. Brain Res.* 6:43-58.

Van der Loos, H. (1967): The history of the neuron. *In: The Neuron.* Hydén, H.,   88
ed. Amsterdam: Elsevier, pp. 1-47.

Van der Loos, H. (1968): Anatomic and physiological consideration. *In: The*   86
Biological Basis of Pediatric Practice. Cooke, R.E., ed. New York: McGraw-Hill,
pp. 1177-1200.

Van der Loos, H. (1972): Autapses in cerebral neocortex. *Anat. Rec.* 172:467.

Van der Loos, H. and Glaser, E.M. (1972): Autapses in neocortex cerebri: synapses   89
between a pyramidal cell's axon and its own dendrites. *Brain Res.* 48:355-360.

Page

Van der Pol, B. (1922): On oscillation hysteresis in a triode generator with two   24
degrees of freedom. *Philos. Mag.* 43:700-719.

Van der Pol, B. and Van der Mark, J. (1928): The heartbeat considered as a   24,71
relaxation oscillation, and an electrical model of the heart. *Philos. Mag.*
6:763-775.

Van Harreveld, A. (1966): *Brain Tissue Electrolytes.* Washington, D.C.: Butterworth, Inc.

Van Harreveld, A. (1966): Extracellular space in the central nervous system. *Proc.
K. Ned. Akad. Wet.* 69:17-21.

Van Harreveld, A. (1970): A mechanism for fluid shifts specific for the central
nervous system. *In: Current Research in Neurosciences, Vol. 10.* Wycis, H.T., ed.
Basel, New York: S. Karger, pp. 62-70.

Van Harreveld, A. (1972): The extracellular space in the vertebrate central nervous   148
system. *In: The Structure and Function of Nervous Tissue.* Bourne, G.H., ed.
New York: Academic Press, pp. 447-511.

Van Harreveld, A. and Fifkova, E. (1970): Glutamate release form the retina during   148
spreading depression. *J. Neurobiol.* 2:13-29.

Van Harreveld, A. and Fifkova, E. (1971): Light- and electron-microscopic changes
in central nervous tissue after electrophoretic injection of glutamate. *Exp. Mol.
Pathol.* 15:61-81.

Van Harreveld, A. and Fifkova, E. (1972): Effects of metabolic inhibitors on the
release of glutamate from the retina. *J. Neurochem.* 19:1439-1450.

Van Harreveld, A. and Fifkova, E. (1973): Mechanisms involved in spreading   149,150
depression. *J. Neurobiol.* 4:375-387.

Van Harreveld, A. and Khattab, F.I. (1967): Changes in cortical extracellular space   150
during spreading depression investigated with the electron microscope. *J. Neurophysiol.* 30:911-929.

Van Harreveld, A. and Khattab, F.I. (1968): Perfusion fixation with glutaraldehyde
and postfixation with osmium tetroxide for electron microscopy. *J. Cell Sci.*
3:579-594.

Van Harreveld, A. and Khattab, F.I. (1969): Changes in extracellular space of the
mouse cerebral cortex during hydroxyadipaldehyde fixation and osmium
tetroxide post-fixation. *J. Cell Sci.* 4:437-453.

Van Harreveld, A., Khattab, F.I., and Steiner, J. (1969): Extracellular space in the
central nervous system of the leech, *Mooreobdella fervida. J. Neurobiol.*
1:23-40.

Van Harreveld, A. and Mahhotra, S.K. (1966): Demonstration of extracellular space
by freeze-drying in the cerebellar molecular layer. *J. Cell Sci.* 1:223-228.

Van Harreveld, A. and Steiner, J. (1970): The magnitude of the extracellular space in electron micrographs of superficial and deep regions of the cerebral cortex. *J. Cell Sci.* 6:793-805.

Volterra, V. (1931): *Lecons sur la Théorie Mathématique de la Lutte pour la Vie.* Paris: Gauthier-Villars.   22

von Euler, C. and Green, J.D. (1960): Activity in single hippocampal pyramids. *Acta Physiol. Scand.* 48:95-109.

Von Tippelskirch, H. (1959): Weitere Konvektionsversuche: der Nachweis der Ringzellen und ihrer Verallgemeinerung. *Beitr. Physik Atmos.* 32:2-22.   16

Vyškočil, F., Kříž, N., and Bureš, J. (1972): Potassium-selective microelectrodes used for measuring the extracellular brain potassium during spreading depression and anoxic depolarization in rats. *Brain Res.* 39:255-259.   127

Walter, D.O. (1971): Alternatives to continuity, observability and passivity in biological modeling. *Math. Biosci.* 11:85-94.

Wang, H.H. and Adey, W.R. (1969): Effects of cations and hyaluronidase on cerebral electrical impedance. *Exp. Neurol.* 25:70-84.   80

Wang, H.H., Tarby, T.J., Kado, R.T., and Adey, W.R. (1966): Periventricular cerebral impedance after intraventricular injection of calcium. *Science* 154:1183-1185.

Ward, A.A., Jr. and Mahnke, J.A. (1960): Standing potential characteristics of the epileptogenic focus. *Trans. Am. Neurol. Assoc.* 85:93-95.

Washburn, A.L. (1956): Classification of patterned ground and review of suggested origins. *Bull. Geol. Soc. Am.* 67:823-866.   22

Watanabe, A. and Bullock, T.H. (1960): Modulation of activity of one neuron by subthreshold slow potentials in another in lobster cardiac ganglion. *J. Gen. Physiol.* 43:1031-1045.

Watanabe, A., Obara, S., and Akiyama, T. (1967): Pacemaker potentials for the periodic burst discharge in the heart ganglion of a stomatopod, *Squilla oratoria. J. Gen. Physiol.* 50:839-862.   73

Waxman, S.G. (1972): Regional differentiation of the axon: A review with special reference to the concept of the multiplex neuron. *Brain Res.* 47:269-288.

Webster, G. (1966): Studies on pattern regulation in hydra. II. Factors controlling hypostome formation. *J. Embryol. Exp. Morphol.* 16:105-122.   65

Wever, R. (1968): Einfluss schwacher elektro-magnetischer Felder auf die circadiane Periodik des Menschen. *Naturwissenschaften* 55:29-32.   140

Whitehead, J.A., Jr. (1971): Cellular convection. *Am. Sci.* 59:444-451.   14,15

	Page

Wiener, N. (1958): Non-linear systems, I. *In: Non-Linear Problems in Random Theory.* Wiener, N., ed. Cambridge, Mass.: M.I.T. Press, pp. 88-96.   71

Wilson, H.R. and Cowan, J.D. (1972): Excitatory and inhibitory interactions in localized populations of model neurons. *Biophys. J.* 12:1-24.   30,74, 75,104,144

Winfree, A.T. (1967): Biological rhythms and the behavior of populations of coupled oscillators. *J. Theor. Biol.* 16:15-42.

Winfree, A.T. (1972): Spiral waves of chemical activity. *Science* 175:634-636.   32,33,57

Wolpert, L. (1969): Positional information and the spatial pattern of cellular differentiation. *J. Theor. Biol.* 25:1-47.   43,64

Woodward, D.L. and Reed, D.J. (1969): Uptake of ^{28}Mg and ^{45}Ca by tissues of magnesium-deficient rabbits. *Am. J. Physiol.* 217:1483-1486.

Zaikin, A.N. and Zhabotinsky, A.M. (1970): Concentration wave propagation in two-dimensional liquid-phase self-oscillating system. *Nature* 225:535-537.   32

Zhabotinsky, A.M. (1967): *In: Oscillatory Processes in Biological and Chemical Systems.* (Symposium of the U.S.S.R. Academy of Science, March 21-26, 1966.) Moscow: Nauka, pp. 149, 181, 199, 252.   30,31, 60

INDEX